Contents

Healthcare Management	1
INDEX	2
Chapter 1	9
Chapter 2	14
Chapter 3	17
Chapter 4	21
Table 2: Managerial positions by organizational setting	23
Chapter 5	26
Chapter 6	32
6.2. In ensuring high results	35
6.3. In the field of talent management	39
6.4.	42
6.5. In terms of change management and creativity	48
6.6. In terms of healthcare reform	52
Chapter 7	55
Table 3: Difference between Managers and Leaders	60
Chapter 9	66
9.1. Model of the Strategic Adaptation	69
Table 4: Different phases of Model of the Strategic Adaptation	73

9.3. The Consumer Sovereignty Model	76
Table 5: Ethical principles of Healthcare with Examples	85
Chapter 11	89
Chapter 12	95
12.1. What is Healthcare Strategic Planning?	96
12.2. Why is Healthcare Strategic Planning Important?	97
Chapter 13	99
Chapter 14	113
14.1. Allied health	116
14.2. Dentistry	119
14.3. Nursing	121
14.4. Pharmacy	123
14.5 Physicians	126
14.6. Physician Assistants	129
Chapter 15	132
	135
Chapter 16	136
Time to Practice	145
Time to Practice	160
The woods are lovely, dark and deep,	177

Preface

It is obvious to ask, why one more book on such a topic. Let me share the story of my journey so far.

I was born in the middle-class family of a small city named Bhagalpur (Bihar, India) famous for its unique silk products and simultaneously recalled for its backward economic status. My father is a retired Professor in agricultural economics. So, literally economics runs in my genes. I grew up hearing about economics jargons from father's mouth while he was discussing with his colleagues or students either on phone or in guest room of our house, located in the big sprawling campus of the agricultural college. Further, I have always loved books and Internet (since a decade) as they help me to quench my thirst of ever-increasing questions. While I was a child, I was sad to know that my state (where I was born) is among the most backward ones and India still a developing economy. Of course, next question used to be how to improve it further.

I was barely 8 years when I could realize my whole family was in big shock, when our dear uncle underwent an open-heart surgery for his chest pain problem. I was sent to a good boarding high school to do my studies, as my father decided to get transferred to a village to stay close to my ageing grandfather and still pursue his job too. During my 16th birthday, I realized that I lost my lovingly elder sister to pulmonary tuberculosis. It really made me determined to pursue medicine at professional level.

During my medicine studies at Bangalore, I further realized that both the ailments are easily preventable. During my medical school days, I really became a big fan of Dr. Devi Shetty who inspite of being a cardiac surgeon is a great entrepreneur too and drew attention for the right reasons. Like every young guy, I wanted to settle down early and earn good money, so I also appeared for MBA entrance exam. I secured 19th all India rank for 2006 Symbiosis Management School entrance test as very few schools offered a specialization in healthcare management. However, some of my friends advised that it is better to pursue such courses after some work experience. Further, the love of clinical field helped me to decide to specialize in cardiology from the Narayana Hrudayalaya Institute of Cardiac Sciences, Bangalore where Dr. Shetty also worked. Here I learnt not only the basics in cardiology but also the unique management principles of my idol. On one side, The Institute offers the best possible success rates (of Cleveland clinic, Massachusetts General Hospital etc.) for the most complex cardiac surgery/interventions at less than fraction of price. He is famously named "Henry Ford of Cardiac Surgery" by Wall Street Journal. He won personal accolades from Mr. David Cameroon during the hospital campus visit and others including Ernst & young, Wall Street Journal, The Economist etc. It further strengthened my views that "As a physician, I can help a few people, however incorporating good management principles; I may be able to help a much bigger society."

During 2008-09 I was able to successfully complete executive program for young professionals from Indian Institute of Management, Kolkata (India) ranked among the best management schools globally.

Further, I obtained my PhD in treatment of most common heart arrhythmia from Maastricht University (The Netherlands) ranked among top 50 global clinical university of world. With time, I am disheartened to realize cardiovascular morbidity and mortality are becoming epidemic not only locally but also globally. During my stint at various academic centres across India, Netherlands, Germany, USA, UK etc I personally felt there is need for better solutions for patient problems. I have actively interacted and attempted to get involved with our managers and clinicians during my stint in India, The Netherlands, USA, and Germany. Our society needs more managers with a medical background as doctors and managers keep focusing on their sphere of work. Our modern world needs more professionals with right mix of medical insights and health economics. Such professionals can understand the intricacies of a hospital or medical industry setup better and still use the expert economic policies for more efficient use of resources.

Even in 21st century, the number of resources used for research and development for a prosthetic limb is much less compared to the research for development of a bumper for a car. Further, although humanity is now aiming to explore for life in other galaxies, but if we talk about the long-term success rate for treatment of most common heart arrhythmia called atrial fibrillation, it is shockingly less than 40 percent.

In 2015, I joined "Master of Science course in Health Economics, Outcomes and Management in Cardiovascular Sciences" from prestigious London School of Economics and political science, UK which is ranked the second best globally among social science universities. The program is collaborated also by European society of Cardiology. The program gave a cardiologist the best possible time to get insights into cardiovascular healthcare and policy related affairs to be able to not just treat the disease but also the root of its origin. Having passed European board examination for cardiac electrophysiologists, I am able to use the knowledge gained from this program for economic analysis and evaluation in field of cardiology especially heart arrhythmias.

This book shares basics of healthcare management to learn the principles of modern epidemiology and health care quality management among the optional subjects. This book will help to share a theoretical and conceptual understanding of health economics, outcomes, research, and healthcare management. The book also shares unique video link to hours of lectures on important related topics for free access to all.

PS: The blank sheets are purposefully provided for readers to take notes and make the book more useful for themselves and society.

© Narendra Kumar, UK
July 2024

No part of this book may be reproduced or transmitted in any form or by any means, without prior permission in writing by the author, or when appropriate, by the publishers of the publications.

Layout: Endra
English editor: Christina

Printed by: Heartbeatsz Academy

Financial support by the Heartbeatsz Academy is gratefully acknowledged

HEALTHCARE
INDUSTRY

LEADERSHIP AND HEALTH ADMINISTRATION

HEALTHCARE MANAGEMENT

BY PROF. DR. NARENDRA KUMAR

Healthcare management is a profession that provides leadership and direction to organizations

Healthcare Management

Narendra Kumar MBBS, MSc, DCC, PhD, FRCP, FACC(USA), FESC, ECES (BE)- level 1 & 2

-Ex Consultant Cardiologist, Bedford University NHS Hospital trust, UK

- Visiting professor Cardiology - EDU(Germany)

-Visiting faculty - Satya Sai Hospital (Raipur), India

-International Education tutor (Royal College of physicians -Edin, UK)

-Program Chair - Cardiology (TAU)

-European Society of Cardiology task force CCG

-Medical Affairs EP -Abbott (USA)

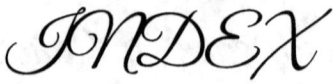

1. A brief introduction..18

2. Administration vs. Healthcare Management.. 24

3. Managerial Requirements and Perspectives..........................28

4. Position and Competency Definition in Management..........................34

5. The Management Job in an Organization's Hierarchy..........................43

6. Managerial responsibilities..48

6.1. In preserving and shaping an organizational culture..........................49

6.2. In ensuring high results..50

6.3. In the field of talent management..52

6.4. In terms of leadership development and succession planning...................53

6.5. In terms of change management and creativity..................................58

6.6. In terms of healthcare reform..60

7. Leadership and Management.. 64

8. The new countervailing force of health administration and professional analysis 70

9. Change of contemporary models in the

3

profession............76

9.1. Model of the Strategic Adaptation............78

9.2. Redesign Model of workplace............80

9.3. The Consumer Sovereignty Model............82

10. Rule of Healthcare Ethics............87

10.1. Step by step instructions to maintain ethics in Healthcare management....89

10.1.1 Arranging Organizational Ethics............91

10.1.2 Advancing Ethics in the Workplace............91

10.1.3 Staff Member Ethics Education............92

10.1.4 Supporting Ethical Behavior............92

10.1.5 Sustaining Free Expression............92

10.1.6 Debilitating Harassment............93

10.1.7 Keeping a Safe Work Environment............93

11. Health care management motivation importance............97

12. Healthcare Strategic

Planning..........105

12.1. What is Healthcare Strategic Planning?............... 106

12.2. Why is Healthcare Strategic Planning Important?............. 106

12.2.1 Communication between all chains has improved

12.2.2 Creating and communicating a vision

12.2.3 Employee motivation and commitment have increased

12.2.4 Authority and transformational leadership

12.2.5 Collaboration and coordination among team members improvement

13. Marketing in the Healthcare Industry...................110

13.1. Marketing Healthcare Services has been around for a long time.........110

13.2. Significant marketing challenges exist for healthcare providers.......... 111

13.3. Definition of production..........111

13.4. The definition of the product....................... 111

13.5. The definition of sale..............111

13.6. The marketing strategy..........112

13.7. The principle of holistic marketing................112

13.8. As a rule, healthcare marketing...112

13.9. The significance of health product marketing................................113

13.10. Effects of Marketing on Healthcare system................................113

14. Healthcare Professions..125

    14.1. Allied health..126

        14.1.1 Schooling/Training

        14.1.2 Clinical Prevention and Population Health Services

        14.1.3 Difficulties/Future Opportunities

    14.2. Dentistry.. 127

        14.2.1 Education/Training

        14.2.2 Clinical Prevention and Population Health Services

        14.2.3 Challenges/Future Opportunities

    14.3. Nursing... 129

        14.3.1 Education/Training

        14.3.2 Clinical Prevention and Population Health Services

        14.3.3 Challenges/Future Opportunities

    14.4.

Pharmacy..........131

    14.4.1 Education/Training

    14.4.2 Clinical Prevention and Population Health Services

    14.4.3 Challenges/Future Opportunities

14.5 Physicians..........132

    14.5.1 Education/Training

    14.5.2 Clinical Prevention and Population Health Services

    14.5.3 Challenges/Future Opportunities

14.6. Physician Assistants..........135

    14.6.1 Education/Training

    14.6.2 Clinical Prevention and Population Health Services

    14.6.3 Challenges/Future Opportunities

15. Video Lectures..........140

16. References..........146

17. Time to Practice - Multiple Choice Question..........154

18. **Brief** **Biodata** 188

The BONUS Chapters

19. Self Care

20. Communication and Counselling

Chapter 1

A brief Introduction

Healthcare management is a growing field with opportunities in both direct and indirect care settings.

Buchbinder and Thompson (2010, pp. 33–34) put it this way:

• Direct care settings are "any organizations that provide direct care to a patient, occupant, or consumer who seeks services from the organization."

• Non-direct care settings are not directly involved in considering individuals who need health administrations; instead, they support people's consideration by providing products and services to direct care settings.

According to the Bureau of Labor Statistics (BLS, 2014), health care management is one of the fastest growing occupations because of the growth and extension of the medical care sector. According to the BLS, medical and healthcare administration directors are expected to grow by 23% between 2012 and 2022, faster than the average for all occupations.

Inpatient and outpatient care facilities need these administrators, with the best opportunities for advancement in management roles occurring in outpatient settings, centers, and doctor practices. Because of the medical clinic's enormous scale, the hospital would need to fill a number of executive roles. The crucial development of organizational circumstances in non-direct care environments, such as therapy companies, pharmacy associations, affiliations, and clinical hardware organizations, is not reflected in these evaluations. These non–direct care environments greatly aid the coordination of consideration associations. Since the number of administrative positions in direct care is expected to grow significantly, it is natural that growth would also occur in administrative positions in non-direct care settings.

Healthcare management is a profession that provides leadership and direction to organizations that deliver individual health administrations, as well as departments, offices, units, or administrations within those organizations. Individuals who need to have an impact on the lives of others will find great rewards and personal satisfaction in health care management. This section provides a comprehensive overview of health care management as a profession. Understanding the roles, responsibilities, and capabilities of health care managers is critical for those considering the profession to make informed decisions about the "fit."

The term "healthcare management" refers to just what the name implies. It's the general manager of a medical facility, such as a clinic or a hospital. A healthcare director is in charge of ensuring that a healthcare facility is operating according to its financial plan, the office's professionals' goals, and the needs of the surrounding community. A person in charge of healthcare services oversees the facility's day-to-day operations.

This person also acts as a spokesperson for the company when providing information to the media. The person in charge of healthcare management frequently collaborates with clinical personnel pioneers on clinical equipment, office budget plans, and planning strategies to ensure the hospital achieves its goals and maintains good relationships with experts, medical caretakers, and office heads. Execution reviews, personnel assumptions, preparation, online media alerts, and billing are things that the healthcare manager decides on.

Healthcare executives are responsible for a variety of tasks. Managers will be in charge of the scheduling of care workers such as nurses and CNAs. They will also ensure that patients receive high-quality treatment. To do so, they should conduct understanding care studies and respond to any patient complaints that arise.

"Healthcare management" is a broad word that encompasses a variety of job titles. Healthcare management degrees are commonly held by clinical chiefs, healthcare administrators, health organizers, and nursing home facilitators. Suppose you can think of healthcare managers as people who work in hospitals or private practice. In that case, they may also work in schools or universities, general health communities, critical care facilities, insurance providers, or drug companies.

Those with healthcare management degrees can need to look at more specialized areas of healthcare management. Health data management is a fantastic model. From hospitals to critical care environments to general practitioner's offices, every type of healthcare practice maintains a data collection of patient health data. A group of experts maintains these data sets. IT experts create the data sets, professionals and staff enter health information, and clinical charting and coding experts ensure that procedures are correctly coded for security.

Someone from the health-care industry has to look at the larger picture and ensure that the databases are up to date. They may be in charge of all aspects of the database. A health information manager, for example, may collaborate with cybersecurity experts to ensure that the database is safe enough to prevent data breaches. They can also collaborate with doctors and nurses to improve treatment and clinic visit documentation. They often evaluate the data collection and documentation process regularly to ensure the databases operate optimally.

At the end of the day, healthcare management practitioners are responsible for overseeing and coordinating healthcare aspects. These administrators ensure that healthcare facilities run smoothly for everyone involved, whether they're managing hospital activities or organizing events in a small private practice.

Chapter 2

Administration vs. Healthcare Management

The phrases as healthcare management and healthcare administration are often used interchangeably, and many believe they mean the same thing. They are two distinct entities.

Healthcare management is in charge of the whole healthcare organization, while healthcare administration is the employees' order. Staffing for a specific division can fall under the purview of the healthcare administration. The healthcare manager, on the other hand, can determine if another representative is required. As a result, healthcare executives are in charge of the corporate side of healthcare organizations.

A healthcare administration will determine the best methods for assisting employees in being proficient at their jobs and understanding the office's treatment. The healthcare manager decides on treatment, staffing levels, and how each division should be run. Healthcare administrators focus on the needs and direction of a hospital or other clinical environment from a 10,000-foot perspective, while overseers concentrate on dealing with the staff to a large degree. In hospitals, healthcare administrators are in charge of hospital-wide issues, while chairpersons are in charge of specific offices.

Even though healthcare management and administration have different responsibilities, they often collaborate, particularly when implementing a successful strategy or innovation changes. In more modest settings (such as private practices), one person may fulfill both the administrative and managerial roles.

Chapter 3

Managerial Requirements and Perspectives

Health-care organizations are complex and diverse, and their existence necessitates that managers delegate power and oversee and coordinate staff. Associations were formed to achieve goals that were outside the reach of any single individual. The scope and complexity of errands performed in administrations' arrangements are so great in health care organizations that a single employee working alone could not keep up with the workload. Furthermore, the critical tasks of developing services in health-care organizations necessitate the integration of a large number of highly specific teaches that must work together continuously.

Organizations require managers to ensure that their activities are performed flawlessly to achieve authoritative goals. Adequate resources, including financial and human resources, are available to assist the organization. Health-care executives are promoted to positions of authority, where they help to influence the organization by making important decisions. Staff enlistment and promotion, securing innovation, administration rises and decreases, and allotment and expenditure of monetary assets are examples of such decisions. Health-care executives' decisions address ensuring that the patient receives the most appropriate, fair, and persuasive administrations possible and the achievement of the manager's desired execution goals. Finally, an individual manager's decisions have an effect on the organization's overall image.

When carrying out different tasks and making decisions, managers must understand two areas (Thompson, 2007). External and internal domains are the names given to these two types of domains.

The external domain refers to external forces, tools, and events that directly impact the organization. Community needs, demographic characteristics, reimbursement from private insurers, and government plans such as the Children's Health Insurance Program (CHIP), Medicare, and Medicaid are among these variables.

The internal domain relates to the issues that managers must deal with regularly, such as ensuring the right number and types of employees, financial results, and care quality. The functioning of the company is reflected in these internal areas, where the manager has the most influence. Maintaining a dual viewpoint necessitates a great deal of balance and commitment on management to make the best decisions.

Managers should think of two domains when running errands and making decisions (Thompson, 2007). These are referred to as external and internal realms, respectively.

On the other hand, the external domain refers to the external effects, properties, and activities that have a significant effect on the organization. Local needs, population characteristics, and repayment from business guarantors and government plans such as the Children's Health Insurance Plans (CHIP), Medicare, and Medicaid are among these factors.

The internal domain refers to the areas of the center that managers must handle on a regular basis, such as ensuring the right number and types of employees, financial execution, and the nature of the treatment. The operation of the association where the manager has the most influence is mirrored in these inward regions. Maintaining the dual perspective necessitates a delicate balance and a concerted effort on the part of management to make sound decisions.

Domains of Health Services Administration

External	Internal
Community demographics	Staffing
Licensure	Budgeting
Accreditation	Quality services
Regulations	Patient satisfaction
Stakeholder demands	Physicians relations
Competitors	Financial performance
Medicare and Medicaid	Technology acquisitions
Managed care organizations	New service development

Table 1: Domains of Health Services Administration

Chapter 4

Position and Competency in Management

As previously stated, management is required to assist in facilitating services provided within health care organizations. Management has been described as the cycle that occurs inside organizations to achieve predetermined goals using human and other resources, including social and specialized capacities and exercises (Longest, Rakich, and Darr, 2000).

Managerial positions by organizational setting	
Organizational setting	Examples of managerial positions
Physician practice	Practice manager
	Director of medical record
	Billing office
Nursing home	Administrator
	Manager, business office
	Director, food services
	Admissions coordinator
	Supervisor, environmental services
Hospital	Chief executive officer
	Vice president, Marketing
	Clinical nurse manager
	Director, revenue management
	Supervisor, maintenance

Table 2: Managerial positions by organizational setting

The term implies that managers collaborate with and through others, performing specialized and relational tasks to achieve the organization's ideal goals and objectives. Others have stated that a manager is someone in the organization who supports and is accountable for at least one other person (Lombardi and Schermerhorn, 2007).

Although most beginning students of health care management will focus on the role of the experienced senior director or lead administration of an organization, it is important to remember that management is carried out by a large number of people who do not have the word "manager" in their job title. Boss, facilitator, and director are only a few of the executive positions in health care organizations.

As they complete the management cycle (Longest et al., 2000), managers develop six management capacities:

Designing: The manager's job entails establishing a direction and determining what needs to be improved. It entails determining requirements and setting implementation goals.

Organizing: This organizational job refers to the organization's overall strategy or a specific division, unit, or administration for which the manager is responsible. Furthermore, it entails assigning specific relations and contact instances. This job entails deciding roles, collaborating on assignments, and disseminating power and responsibility.

Staffing: This role refers to the acquisition and retention of human resources. It also refers to the various processes and methods used to create and maintain the labor force.

Controlling: This task entails inspecting personnel exercises and execution and devising appropriate activities for a corrective action to improve execution.

Coordinating: The focus of this position is on establishing an organization through effective management, subordinate motivation, and communication.

Decision maker: This position is fundamental to all of the previously listed management capabilities, and it entails making viable decisions based on the consideration of options' benefits and drawbacks.

The manager would require a few skills to fulfil these responsibilities. The core competencies of a viable manager, according to Katz (1974), include logical, specialized, and relational skills. The word competency refers to a condition in which a person possesses the necessary or satisfactory abilities or characteristics to perform specific tasks (Ross, Wenzel, and Mitlyng, 2002).

These can be defined as follows:

Academic skills are those that have the ability to fundamentally break down and address difficult problems. Models: A manager leads an inquiry into the best way to provide some assistance or agrees on a method to reduce tolerant objections to food service.

Those abilities that demonstrate aptitude or capacity to perform a specific work role are referred to as specialized abilities. Models: A manager develops and implements a new motivational force remuneration scheme for his or her employees, or prepares and implements changes to a PC-based staffing model.

Relational skills enable a manager to communicate with and work well with others, whether they be colleagues, supervisors, or subordinates. Models: A boss informs a worker whose presentation is below expectation or conveys the optimal presentation amount for assistance for the next fiscal year to subordinates.

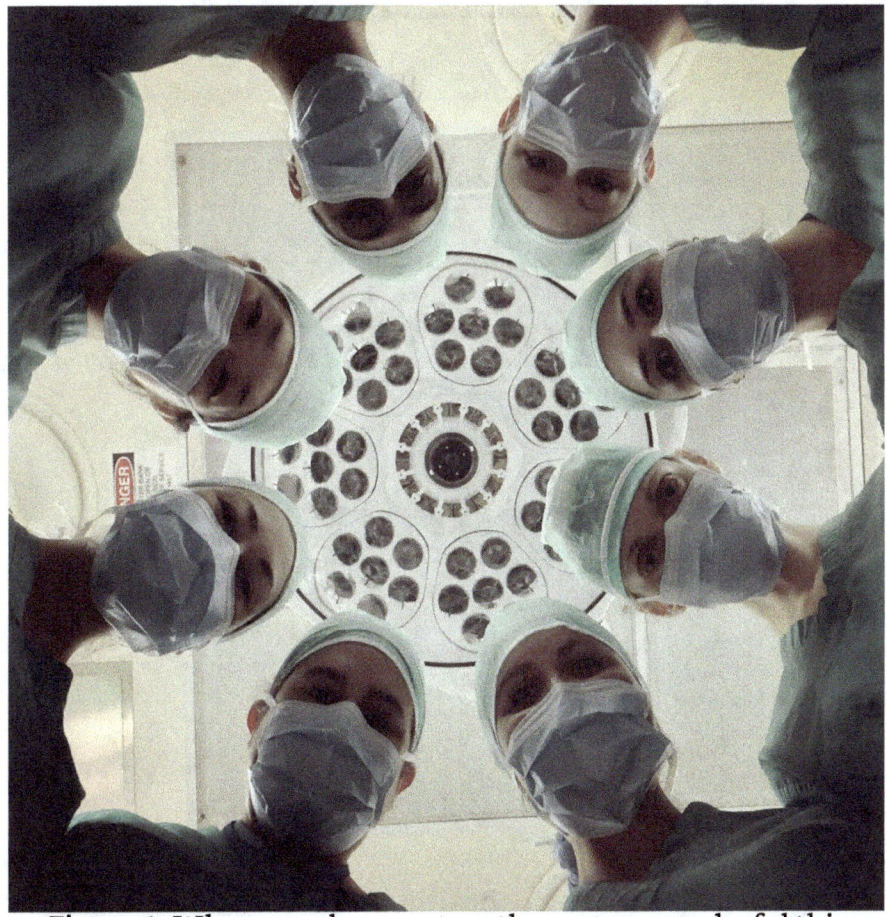

Figure 1: When people come together, more wonderful things happen together.

Chapter 5

The Management Job in an Organization's Hierarchy

Management positions in health care organizations are not limited to the top levels; due to the scale and complexity of many health care organizations, management positions can be found across the organization. There are management roles at the lower, middle, and upper levels; the latter is referred to as senior management.

The hierarchy system of management means that positions, or powers, are assigned in descending order within the organization. Lower-level managers have less power than higher-level managers, whose scope of responsibility is much greater. A VP of Patient Care Services in a hospital, for example, can be responsible for a number of different functional areas, such as nursing, analytic imaging administrations, and testing facility administrations; on the other hand, a Medical Records Overseer—a lower-level position—is solely responsible for the task of patient clinical records.

Furthermore, a director of the Environmental Services office may be in charge of a small housekeeping staff whose responsibilities are limited to a specific area of the organization. Some managerial roles, for example, are line manager positions because the manager supervises various representatives; others are staff manager positions because they complete work and motivate their subordinates. They may not, however, routinely supervise others.

In terms of needed skills or experience, managerial positions vary as well. A few positions necessitate extensive knowledge of various significant territories as well as relevant job experience, while others are better suited to entry-level managers with little or no experience. A successful hierarchical architecture is the most well-known authoritative structure for health care organizations. A pyramid-shaped progression characterizes the task being played and the key management positions allotted to such roles as the key trademark.

The formal structure will be determined by the size and complexity of the particular health administration association. For example, larger organizations—such as large community hospitals, hospital systems, and academic clinical centers—are likely to have complex vertical structures representing varying levels of regulatory control. Because of the large number of administrations provided and the wide variety of authoritative and support resources required to enable the delivery of clinical services, this structure is critical.

Other characteristics of this useful structure include a strict hierarchy of leadership and revealing lines, which ensure that communication and task and project evaluation are performed in a direct and controlled environment. Explicit job groups, simple announcing, and responsibility lines are among the main features of this structure.

Health care organizations have adopted other authoritative designs, usually in conjunction with a functional structure: grid, or group-based, models, and administration line management models. A rugged utilitarian construction, according to the lattice model, can limit the association's adaptability to do the job, and different orders' skill is required on a continuous basis.

When practical personnel, such as nursing and rehabilitation faculty, are assigned to a specific program, such as geriatrics, this is an example of the lattice technique. The report is sent automatically to the geriatrics division's programed head. Another model is where clinical and administrative personnel are assigned to a department that is tasked with evaluating new administrations under the supervision of an advertisement or business development manager. In both models, management would guide employees who were not directly under their authority. Improved parallel communications and administration teamwork, as well as pooled information, are all advantages of this structure. A manager is assigned to head a specific clinical helpline and is responsible for personnel, asset acquisition, budgeting, and monetary control for the various administrations provided within that help line. Cardiology, oncology (cancer), women's administrations, physical rehabilitation, and social health are all common administration lines (emotional well-being). Administration lines may be established within a single organization or through subsidiary organizations, such as within a hospital system where administrations are provided at a few exceptional partnered facilities (Boblitz and Thompson, 2005).

When compared to other management models, a few providers have discovered that the helpline management model for specific clinical administrations has resulted in various benefits, including reduced costs, higher quality of treatment, and greater patient satisfaction (Duffy and Lemieux, 1995).

The assistance line management model is typically implemented within a company that is linked to a valuable structure. One or more service lines may receive special attention and additional resources from the organization.

Management's main focus

At three levels, effective health-care management entails exercising professional judgement and skills, as well as completing the previously listed administrative capacities:

- Individually
- Within a unit/group
- Through the whole association

Above all, the person manager should be able to properly handle himself. This entails managing time, data, space, and materials; being attentive and follow-through with colleagues, managers, and customers; and maintaining a positive attitude and high levels of motivation. Maintaining a current understanding of strategic practices and important health-care management problems.

Managing yourself, according to Drucker (2005), entails understanding your qualities, how you play out, where you should be, and what you should contribute, as well as taking responsibility for your relationships. Managing yourself often entails developing and applying appropriate advanced, relational, and measured abilities and skills, as well as being comfortable with them, in order to effectively progress to the next level—that of regulating others.

The unit/group level is the second focal point of management. At this stage, the manager's ability to handle others requires ensuring that the work is completed properly. If you're a senior director, a mid-level boss, or a manager, you'll be "regulating" those in your assigned position. This responsibility entails allocating job errands, surveys, and task changes, observing and auditing individual execution, and completing the management capacities outlined previously to ensure excellent administration delivery. This central zone is where the real work is done. The officeholder on the administrator is responsible for shaping the show of individual employees, and execution reflects the cooperation of the chief and the delegate. The focal point of management at this level recognizes the interdependencies among employees' assignments as well as the close teamwork required to ensure that work is completed proficiently and adequately.

The hierarchical management center is the third management center. This core territory reflects how managers can work together as part of a larger organization to ensure consistent implementation and authoritative practicality. The effectiveness of the organization is contingent on its members completing their tasks, and effective collaboration is required to ensure that this occurs. The breadth of clinical and nonclinical activities inside a healthcare organisation necessitates that unit managers collaborate closely with other unit managers to provide support. For development, data sharing, concerted effort, and correspondence are essential. Following the entirety, the order looks to each administered unit's dedication. Individual managers' contributions to the association's overall presentation—in terms of various execution estimates such as cost, efficiency, fulfilment, and access—are substantial and uncertain.

Chapter 6

Managerial

Responsibilities

6.1. In preserving and shaping an organizational culture

Each company has its own distinct culture, which is defined by the shared convictions, mentalities, and behaviors of its employees.

Organizational culture is typically described as the "character," "personality," and "experience" of organizational life, i.e., what the organization "is" (Scott, Mannion, Davies, and Marshall, 2003). The management community defines, forms, and supports culture, which recommends the status quo. Both managers play a role in shaping the culture of a healthcare institution and in exercising significant authority to preserve and often alter the culture. The qualities, mission, and vision of an organization form its culture.

Values are standards that an organization believes are well-suited to the organization's motivation, goals, and day-to-day operations. Embraced principles guide the organization's activities and provide requirements for quality assistance and development.

The organization's purpose is its basic reason for being, or what it seeks to achieve.

The organization's vision defines its desired future state and represents how it wants to be known and regarded in the future. The organizational main arranging measure results in proclamations of qualities, purpose, and vision. These assertions are disseminated widely within the organisation and to the surrounding community, and they help to shape the organization's critical and operational activities.

Organizations are increasingly establishing tacit standards or codes of conduct for all employees to obey (Studer, 2003). These conduct guidelines correspond to the qualities, mission, and vision. Setting assumptions for staff behavior, showing the conduct, estimating staff execution, and enhancing staff execution are all basic responsibilities of managers in the supervision of conduct norms. Mid-level and lower-level administrators play a critical role in the culture's adoption and adoption within the enterprise. By expressing assumptions through their practices, they express desired practices and support culture. Managers must ensure adequate administration degrees by their employees by communicating assumptions and providing inward client assistance to their staff and managers, for example, in a client assistance or patient center estimation. Managers may also inspect representative execution and collaborate with workers to enhance execution to gauge and evaluate worker compliance with organizational qualities and rules of behavior.

6.2. In ensuring high results

At the end of the day, the manager's job is to ensure that the unit, operation, division, or organisation he or she leads performs well. What exactly does "high execution" imply? To achieve execution, one must value the benefits of identifying and achieving goals and priorities for the unit/service and organization's work. Goals and objectives are desired end points for action that represent the organization's critical and organizational headings.

They are specific, quantifiable, important, and chronologically ordered. Individual unit objectives and goals should reflect the organization's overall requirements and assumptions, since, as the reader can see, all elements are working together to achieve high levels of overall organizational execution.

Studer (2003) sees the company as a waiting room for performance, with well-known mainstays of greatness serving as a structure for its specific goals. Individuals (representatives, patients, and doctors), operation, efficiency, capital, and creation are the columns.

Griffith (2000) refers to high-performing organizations as title organizations, implying that they aspire to excel in a variety of but important aspects of execution. Griffith goes on to describe the need for "title steps" in each of the following areas: administration and key management; clinical efficiency, including patient loyalty; clinical organisation (caregivers); financial planning; planning and advertising; data services; HR; and plant and supplies. The organisation should build up proportions of desired execution for each title period in order to guide the organisation. Drug errors, diligent inconveniences, customer satisfaction, staff turnover rates, worker satisfaction, market share, benefit advantage, and income growth are examples of interventions. As a result, individual divisions, departments, and programs will set goals and conduct drills to resolve key performance indicators.

Finally, the administrator's job ensures that these goals are reached by using the recently reviewed management capabilities. Ginter, Swayne, and Duncan (2002) developed a control interaction for managers that depicts five main steps in the exhibition management measure: set destinations, measure execution, compare execution and objectives, determine reasons for deviation, and make a corrective move. The duty of management is to ensure that the exhibition is maintained or, if necessary, enhanced.

Partners, such as contingency plans, state and national governments, and shopper marketing groups, anticipate and, in most cases, demand sufficient levels of implementation from health-care organizations. These meetings must ensure that resources are provided in a secure, beneficial, low-effort, and high-quality environment.

The Joint Commission (formerly JCAHO) has established minimum standards for health-care office activities to ensure consistency, the National Committee for Quality Assurance (NCQA) has established standards for calculating health-plan execution, and the Centers for Medicare and Medicaid Services (CMS) has established a website that considers hospital execution as well as various basic metrics. CMS has also provided impetus to health-care organizations by paying for clinical care based on proportions rather than care resulting from never events, i.e., stunning health outcomes that should never occur in a health-care setting, such as the wrong site for a medical procedure (e.g., some unacceptable leg) or hospital-acquired diseases (Agency for Healthcare Research and Quality, n.d.).

Similarly, health backup initiatives have implemented pay-for-execution systems for health care organizations based on various quality and customer service metrics.

In addition to meeting the detailing requirements of the aforementioned organizations, several health-care organizations now use various techniques for estimating and disclosing the exhibition estimation measure. Traditional methods include developing and deploying dashboards or adjusted scorecards that take into account a quick translation of organizational performance across various main metrics (Curtright, Stolp-Smith, and Edell, 2000; Pieper, 2005).

These strategies are used by the senior organisation to assess and communicate the overall organization's execution to the overseeing board and other key stakeholders. Different managers use these strategies to profile their exhibition at the division, section, or service level. These metrics are often used to evaluate managers' performance and are taken into account by the chief's boss when making decisions about remuneration, advancements, increased or decreased responsibilities, training and development, and, if necessary, termination or reassignment.

6.3. In the field of talent management

Management should have the appropriate number and styles of strongly persuaded members to adequately dominate the core areas of management and complete the necessary management capacities in the field of talent management. Fundamentally, health-care organizations need to fill positions, and it is now generally acknowledged that high-performing health-care organizations need superior human performance.

Several eyewitnesses have argued that health-care organizations should view their members as important resources from which they can benefit (Becker, Huselid, and Ulrich, 2001). HR management has been largely replaced by talent management in many health-care organizations. Rather than focusing on filling a vacancy, the emphasis has moved to learning and retaining the skills needed to do the job well (Huselid, Beatty, and Becker, 2005). Managers are now focused on efficiently managing capability and labor force issues as a result of the connection to organizational execution (Griffith, 2009).

After enlistment, managers are worried with recruiting and retaining talented entertainers. Many health-care organizations are forming high-inclusion organizations that recognize and address employee issues through their employment and the broader work climate (Becker et al., 2001). One of the fundamental duties of a manager's inability management is advance representative commitment, which represents the staff's motivation and obligation to contribute to the business. Managers use a variety of programs to encourage and maintain representative commitment to producing and preserving exceptional entertainers. Traditional strategies such as providing training, providing initiative implementation plans, identifying worker needs, and estimating representative satisfaction through commitment studies are among them. Other strategies include providing training, particularly in clinical and specialized fields, and empowering position advancement. Easy strategies for managing representative relations and interaction include performing periodic worker audits, soliciting representative criticism, directing rounds and worker groups, offering worker idea services, and other techniques.

6.4.

In terms of leadership development and succession planning,

Since health-care organizations are inherently unpredictable and face challenges from both within and outside, managers' leadership skills at all levels have become increasingly relevant.

Effective organizations that have a high level of organizational execution need solid pioneers (Squazzo, 2009). Senior executives are crucial in ensuring that all managers have the expertise and skills they need to provide effective leadership and achieve the required levels of organizational execution. Senior management is also crucial to growth, as they must ensure that opportunities at the mid- and upper levels of the organisation are filled with capable pioneers such that retirements, takeoffs, and inventions are all filled with capable pioneers. As a consequence, developing future pioneers through leadership growth activities and participating in progression preparation is one of the most significant roles of managers.

In most health-care organizations, leadership development programs have a few basic organizational services aimed at enhancing administrative staff's leadership skills and abilities.

Educational mediations and skill-building exercises aimed at strengthening people's leadership skills are referred to as leadership development (Kim and Thompson, 2012; McAlearney, 2005). Via career development and planning, such programs not only help to improve leadership skills and practices, but they also help to ensure organizational capacity and culture (Burt, 2005). Managers who promote leadership development provide their workers with specialized and emotional support through a range of leadership development programs, such as:

Training and leadership development on a number of important points within an officially assigned program, using standardized learning and competency-based testing in a variety of settings, media, and regions (Kim and Thompson, 2012)

Courses in management and leadership: Exact courses delivered in person, online, or in a hybrid format include didactic training (Garman, 2010; Kim and Thompson, 2012)

Tutoring: The organizations systematic processes for pairing up young pioneers with mid-level and senior chiefs to help them learn and develop (Garman, 2010; Landry and Bewley, 2010)

Self-improvement education: These organized organizational endeavors, which are typically reserved for upper-level executives, help to improve execution by molding perspectives and behavior and concentrating on close-to-home ability growth (Garman, 2010; Scott, 2009)

Occupation broadening: Providing expanded tasks, formative positions, and unconventional ventures to people in order to develop leadership skills and advance within the business is known as occupation broadening (Fernandez-Aaroz, 2014; Garman, 2010; Landry and Bewley, 2010)

360-degree execution criticism: A multisource feedback approach in which a single staff member or administrator receives an appraisal of execution from a few key people (e.g., colleagues, supervisors, various administrators, and subordinates) in terms of execution and growth opportunities (Garman, 2010; Landry and Bewley, 2010)

Projects aimed at developing leaders have shown positive results. When leadership growth is linked to organizational-wide critical needs, such as improving labor force skills and nature, improving organizational efficiency in instructional activities, and lowering staff turnover and related costs, for example, health structures reveal benefits such as improving labor force skills and nature, improving organizational efficiency in instructional activities, and lowering staff turnover and related costs (McAlearney, 2005). Furthermore, hospitals with leadership development programs have higher patient rates, higher occupancy, higher net patient income, and a higher gross profit margin than hospitals without these projects (Thompson and Kim, 2013).

Health-care leadership development programs have been

linked to a greater emphasis on representative growth and transformation, improved employee retention, and a more focused outlook on vital organizational needs, according to reports (McAlearney, 2010). Finally, within a single health system, a leadership development program resulted in more powerful segments of the overall sector, lower staff turnover, and improved center quality controls (Ogden, 2007). Nonetheless, the expense of designing and implementing leadership development programs is one of the most important drawbacks (Squazzo, 2009).

Because of the serious nature of health care organizations and the need for highly motivated and gifted members, managers are put to the test when it comes to planning for their organizations.

The process of ensuring that workers can advance in management roles within the company to replace those who retire or leave for other opportunities is referred to as progression planning. Because of the large number of Baby Boomer (CEO) retirements anticipated, progression preparation has recently been emphasized at the executive level of businesses (Burt, 2005). CEOs and other top executives are searching for and maintaining leadership talent within their organizations that can take responsibility and carry forward the organization's essential work in order to keep the emphasis on high execution.

To meet leadership growth criteria, health-care organizations are currently focused on a few practices. To begin with, junior management tutoring with senior management support has been marketed as a good way to train future health-care pioneers (Rollins, 2003). Tutoring means proving to coaches that their efforts are helpful to the organisation (Finley, Ivanitskaya, and Kennedy, 2007). Several eyewitnesses recommend offering several guides in order to capture the required degree of skill, expertise, interest, and connections in order to advance one's career (Broscio and Scherer, 2003). Coaching center-level managers for promotion as they move to their new positions will help them prepare for future chief leadership roles (Kubica, 2008).

Traditional leadership development programs are a second choice for planning advancement. These programs concentrate on people's clear ranges of abilities and evaluate their fit for particular positions, such as vice president or chief operating officer, in order to recognize management potential in an organisation (COO). Conducting annual talent surveys is one way to do this, as it helps to build a pool of existing workers that could be outstanding candidates for further leadership growth and ability reinforcement through the use of advancement plans. Many health-care organizations are implementing formal programs aimed at high-potential people (Burt, 2005). Thompson and Kim (2013) estimate that 48% of community hospitals offer a leadership development program. According to McAlearney (2010), approximately half of all hospital systems in the United States have a top-level leadership development program. In any case, a range of health-care organizations have launched programs aimed at strengthening leadership across the board, not just at the top. All managers are expected to take part in these activities in order to develop their management and leadership skills, as well as the company's performance.

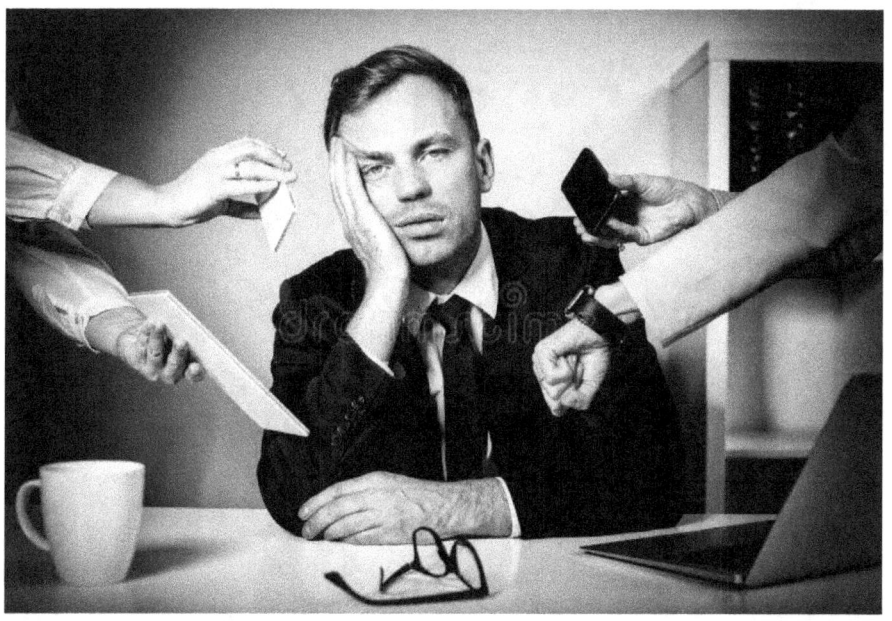

6.5. In terms of change management and creativity

Because of the rapid pace of change in the health-care sector and the complexity of healthcare organizations, the director plays a critical role in guiding growth and implementing change management. Organizations that provide health care facilities cannot remain stagnant. The natural forces discussed earlier in this section emphasize the need for organizations to respond to and adapt to these external influences. Furthermore, achieving and maintaining high execution performance or results improves organizational architecture and cycles. Managers are also encouraged to welcome change in order to recognize innovative ways to enhance quality and provide treatment in a viable and sustainable manner.

Advancement and change management are intricately linked, despite their exceptional capabilities. Hamel (2007) depicts the growth of management and the expansion of operations. Management creation is concerned with the organization's management measures, such as the procedures and schedules that determine how management is regularly guided. Within interchanges, job assessment, project management, and planning and development are examples of these methods.

Surprisingly, organizational development pays attention to the organization's financial metrics. Client treatment, provisioning and inventory network shifts, care management across personnel, and innovation and utilization of clinical procedures and methods are all examples of cycles in the health care environment. The acquisition of data and clinical products, such as electronic clinical/health records, or another gadget or method, such as a mechanical medical procedure or new meds, is an example of underlying operational growth (Staren, Braun, and Denny, 2010).

To be trend-setters in management, managers must have specific skills. These skills include proactively improving the company by considering methods to change management and organizational practices. It also provides the opportunity to put these innovative practices to the test and assess their efficacy. Similarly, an employer should promote the recruitment and promotion of employees who value innovation and development.

It is critical to have creative clinical and authoritative personnel when implementing organizational growth. A culture of advancement is dependent on employees who generate ideas for organizational improvement. The chief plays a crucial role in establishing a creation culture that underpins the thought era. Recent research into creative and innovative companies has discovered that pioneers must rely on all employees to work together by supporting one another and participating in a powerful cycle of seeking and giving criticism, ideas, and assistance (Amabile, Fisher, and Pillemer, 2014). There are a few barriers to progression that have been identified. These impediments include a lack of a development community that promotes thinking era, a lack of leadership in advancement efforts, and high costs of implementing innovative changes (Harrington and Voehl, 2010). In addition, formal principles and guidelines, professional norms, and management structures can stifle development (Dhar, Griffin, Hollin, and Kachnowski, 2012).

Finally, everyday needs and inactivity, which cause managers to focus on schedules and daily errands, restrict staff capacity to be creative, engage in disclosure, and build thoughts (Dhar et al., 2012). Organizational change, also known as change management, is related to but distinct from progression. Organizational reform is a systematic management approach to enhancing the organization's performance and appearance. Change management needs information on execution flaws. Managers should review their practical exercises and execution on a regular basis, making adjustments to the work structure and cycles as needed to enhance execution (Thompson, 2010).

Managing organizational change has become a major responsibility for administrators and a necessary skill for health-care executives (Buchbinder and Thompson, 2010).

Managing the interaction of change within health-care organizations is critical because properly and effectively managing change will lead to better organizational execution. Nonetheless, change is difficult, and the change cycle creates both resistance and support for the change. Longest et al. advocated for a cycle model of progress management (2000).

This sensible, issue-based model identifies four important steps in consciously identifying and managing the change interaction:

• Recognizable evidence of the need for change,

• Anticipating and implementing the change,

• Executing and evaluating the change

There are a few main management skills that healthcare executives must possess in order to effectively navigate transition inside their organizations. According to Thompson (2010), managers should: • Embrace change and be a change specialist;

• Implement a change management strategy;

• Effectively overcome change resistance and protection;

• Use change management to make the company more creative and successful in the future; and

• Recruit personnel and develop a progression plan as a result of progress management.

6.6. In terms of healthcare reform

As previously stated in this section, managers should consider both their external and internal areas when assessing their management capabilities and undertakings. One of the most important aspects of navigating the outside environment is to be knowledgeable about health strategy issues that affect health services agencies and health care delivery at the state and federal levels. This is particularly true for senior executives. This knowledge is critical for influencing policy in a confident manner that will assist the company in avoiding any negative consequences.

Maintaining awareness of health-care policy discussions, participating in strategy consultations, and sharing information when necessary would enable health-care management voices to be heard. Since health care is such a well-known but contentious topic in the United States today, reforms in health-care delivery will most likely emanate from administrative and strategy steps at the state and federal levels. For example, the Patient Protection and Affordable Care Act, which was signed into law in 2010 as a major health-care reform initiative, has had substantial implications for health-care organizations in terms of patient volumes, reimbursement for currently uninsured patients, and the advancement of population health and esteem-based purchasing. Cuts in Medicare repayment and expansions in disclosing prerequisites are two recent government strategy shifts.

State administrative changes around the country have an impact on Medicaid and the Children's Health Insurance Program repayments, office and staff licensure, declaration of need rules for capital expenditures and office and service developments, and state requirements on commanded health benefits and adjusted repayments for safeguarded people, all of which have an impact on the services provided by health care organizations.

Managers should strive to keep their knowledge current in order to comprehend and influence health policy. Person picking up, organizing with friends within and outside of their organizations, and participating in professional affiliations such as the American College of Healthcare Executives and the Medical Group Management Association will all help to cultivate this. These and other groups screen health strategy conversations and supporters for the benefits of their affiliations at the state and federal levels. The data gathered as a result of these endeavor can be used to develop health plans that meet the needs of healthcare executives.

Chapter 7

Leadership and Management

There must be leaders and managers in any business setting. Both are not necessarily the same people. Managers might be good leaders, and leaders might be better leaders. In medical services, this is particularly critical to perceive due to the requirement for both. Medical care is special because it is a help industry that relies upon an enormous number of profoundly prepared staff.

An ambulatory care center, a company of insurance, a care facility center, and medical devices, must keep the organization working. Managers and leaders also play an essential role in running the organization in the forward direction. Managers and leaders also maintain current issues and operations in an organization. Acceptable business practices also help in managing and leading the organization.

As a rule, leaders focus on external matters, while the manager focuses on the internal organization's concerns. Even though they should be sure, their medical services office is working appropriately. Leaders, in general, invest most of their energy and time in collaborating and lining up with outside bunches that can profit their organizations (accomplices, local area, sellers) or impact them (government, public organizations, media).

There is a hybrid among managers and leaders across the different regions. However, a qualification stays for specific obligations and duties. Usually, the organization's best individual (e.g., Chief Executive Officer, Administrator, Director) has full and extreme responsibility.

The current conditions might direct this kind of leader by the organization. A good leader is the one who characterizes persistence and vision and adjusts individuals, developments, and qualities that might be required. The leader in an organization connects with the individuals across disciplines ranked offices and locales, which might be fundamental. A few managers will answer the leaders at whichever type of surfaces they work (e.g., Chief Nursing Officer, Physician Director, Chief Information Officer).

These managers can be leaders in their regions. Their focus will be more on the internal organization's activities. The operational heads of the organization are managers. Together, these three kinds of leaders/supporters produce a related authority framework that will demonstrate all the more high acting in the current medical care field (Maccoby, Norman, Norman, and Margolies, 2013).

Leaders have a specific arrangement of capabilities that require more groundbreaking than those of managers. In an organization, leaders need to set inventiveness or directions. They should have the option to stimulate their employees and investors so the business proceeds to exist and, ideally, flourish in times of progress.

No industry is as robust as medical services, with quick-change because of the framework and government guidelines' intricacy. Leaders are expected to keep the unit on course and move around hindrances, similar to a commander telling his boat adrift. Administrators and managers should keep an eye on the current business and ensure that the staff follows legitimate systems and meets set-up targets and objectives. They need an alternate arrangement of capabilities.

	Managers	**Leaders**
Focus	Transactional	Transformational
	Meeting objectives and delegating tasks	Developing a vision and a way forward
Priority	Work	People
	Goal is to get things done, task management	Care about you and want you to succeed; behavioral focus
Team	Subordinates	Followers
	Lead through	Lead through

		authority and task management; telling	inspiring and circles of influence; involve & motivate
	Ethics	Do right things	Do the right things
		Follow the rules and maintain status	Shape the culture and act with integrity; break rules if needed

Table 3: Difference between Managers and Leaders

Chapter 8

The new countervailing forces of health administration and professional analysis

More than 25 years prior, there was an acknowledgment of the potential for the medication to "keep a self-misdirecting vision of objectivity and firm quality of its information and the ethics of its individuals [leading] to insularity and an egotism about its main goal on the planet" (Freidson 1970). During the 1990s, coordinated medication, nursing, and allied sciences' health professionals discover their capacity to fill in as "labor market shelters" (Freedman 1976; Freidson 1994) to impact self-seeking just as the interests of different professions progressively reduced. Emergency clinics, HMOs, and the individuals who denote patients are in a situation to move the overall influence and clinical parts among diverse medical care professions (Begun and Lippincott 1993; Schneller, Hood-Szivek, and Hughes 1994).

Few health care professionals feel a complete disassociation with their working environment due to expansion. Without a doubt, a period where claims for limited or enhancing power or jurisdiction cases are troublesome (Akers 1968).

In hospitals, multi-skilled practitioners have been shifted. E.g., inhalation therapists find that parts of their work are progressively performed by nonprofessionals (Hyde and Fottler 1995).

Head administrators of health services are no outsiders to the thought processes related to labor force change. In territories where doctors and medical caretakers are in excess, health professionals are treated as business contributions to the "product" called health care. In such cases, experts experience argumentative relations with supplier associations (Begun and Lippincott 1993).

An explanation of changes forced through the rearrangement of health professionals' work is that the idea of "workforce reform" is a codeword utilized by administrators for shifting work to the most reduced expense, yet qualified, supplier. The substitute clarification is that labor force change is essential for a rational and balanced process guaranteeing excellent results and outcomes.

Care-managed advanced systems like Kaiser Permanente model staffing determine the equilibrium of doctors, doctor assistants, nurses, and attendants for clinical administrations dependent on the serving population's size.

The administrators should perceive that while a few clinicians dread that, they will lose employment opportunities. Professionals standards and protocols of clinics, once grown inside by rehearsing clinicians, will probably be forced by nonprofessionals or nonpracticing clinicians who have become expert information supervisors (Hafferty and McKinlay 1993).

The new procedures of reshaping work's dependent on such investigations may weaken the "action orientation" part of expert work: "The main objective reason of experts towards quick action is instead of depicting what is continually making decisions about the suitable action course in a given circumstance" (Cervero 1989). The media have recognized these forces and started to screen them into secular culture.

The Economist's (1994) article has recommended that "the fate of specialists looks grim. To improve proficiency, another type of medical care managers are meddling in verdicts that were at one time the save of the medical profession."

The problem range is flexible to clinics' protocols, and the impacts of these instructions have not been established yet. There is a developing belief that the same force can plot medical care work that shapes the work in producing and different parts of the service sector. The health profession's organization around set up authorities or auction domains and "proficient standards" (Freidson 1973). It has truly given significant "countervailing forces" (Light 1993; Johnson 1972; and Larson 1977; Galbraith 1956) to guarantee that changing conditions in the construction of medical services conveyance don't compromise the activity direction of expert work (Schon 1982).

There is an expanded dread that the labor force upgrade as a procedure-related to managed care. It is hired to restrict access to expensive administrations through watchmen "instead of as far as planning crafted by semi-self-governing experts, explaining lines of power and assisting patients by arguing administrations and trained professional specialists and services" (Geretis 1993).

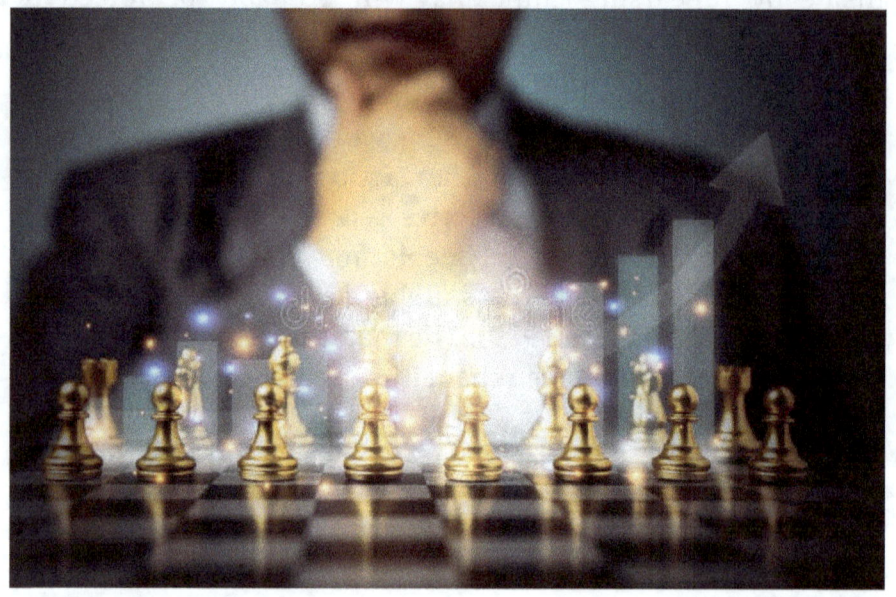

Institutional medical services buyers and vertically incorporated frameworks comprise new countervailing forces and take steps to end the medical profession supremacy (Light 1993) and the energy that nursing has had in planning bedside system of care frameworks. In this climate, the medical services manager should identify the role that administration and management can play as a countervailing force to guarantee an environment in which technical information is utilized to the patient's advantage.

Managers who identify the satisfaction of the patient have prolonged effects on their organization's feasibility. Improving the healthiness status of the systems and communities should guarantee that their clinical staff is coordinated to accomplish payers, patients, and societies. While it isn't sure that doctors' employment and the upgrade and decrease of expert work for patient consideration essentially diminishes the nature of medical services and supplier fulfillment (Wolinsky and Marder 1993; Stamps and Cruz 1994), there is proof that the reengineering of medication to serve roles that rise above customary clinical interests, can prompt more extensive decay of medical care system (Field 1993; Freidson 1994).

Chapter 9

Change of contemporary models in the profession

Change in the work environment dominates conversations

about clinical work and experts.

Andrew Abbott (1988) first discussed this idea in the paper, describes workers of health care as existing inside a "system of the profession" (SOP) in which the main principle is securing the jurisdiction that is employed by profession to ensure their place in the labor division of the medical profession. The SOP model distinguishes the trouble in changing the professionals' jurisdictions whenever they have been set up. The occupations are viewed as existing inside a work division that is liable to change, especially in information development, shortage, overflow of staff, or intrusion by elective/substitute profession. By specifying the formal and casual elements of expert life, the SOP model gives the establishment to appreciate the distinctions in staffing patterns among organizations and the potential for overseeing proficient work in a time of marketplace change. Another model, progressed by Begun and Lippincott (1993), expands on prior research in essential voting public administration to propel a "strategic adaptation model" (SA) for the professionals.

The S.A. model resists that professions through the principal associations, engagement in various activities, or securing their position in the changing system. The S.A. model alarms us to the expert world dynamics: Administrators, regulators, and buyers endeavor to shape the professions to address the medical environment's varying needs. A third model, "redesigning patient care" (RPC), centers around the service needs of the patient within various units of an organization (e.g., the "hospital floor" or administration) as the beginning stage for comprising the division of work.

The RPC model at that point applies current day board standards, including the ideas of teamwork, proficiency, work plan, job design, and total quality administration, to forming and assigning work inside hospitals and other medical services organizations. PRC's perspective is the industrial principles logical application (Schneller, Hood-Szivek, and Hughes 1994) to medical services labor force upgrade.

The last model we will survey is marked "consumer sovereignty" (C.S.) and emphasis the role of people inside communities as the foremost determinant of expert administrations and expert work. This model assumes a genuinely wide variety in variations and requirements for medical care administrations and projects participatory profession, instead of a dominant role in the assurance and conveyance of health administrations. Before specifying the models, it is significant that there might be various essential highlights or covering worries inside the multiple models. Each model's great part has substantial implications for the profession's future.

9.1. Model of the Strategic Adaptation

The S.A. model recommends that the conditions that upheld the U.S.'s health professionals have gone through quick change and prompted the callings' destabilization.

The key elements are:

- Expansion of the occupational customer base has paved the way for demographic trends.
- The specialized knowledge and technology claim that the profession's research infrastructure generates the power of grounding professionals. It accesses to the profession.
- Abundant financing has offered an approach to direct the care and a controlled progression of dollars.
- The professionals of health care once attributed a significant degree of regard and trust has offered an approach to doubt of experts' intentions.
- The formal government's protection and support are no longer guaranteed as the govt itself. It acts to shape the development, practiced guidelines, support competition, and discourage licensing the professionals.

While populace development in the past may have established an environment that created an interest for health experts' administrations (Begun and Lippincott 1993), the scant asset in the present medical care framework is the patient (Schneller, Hood-Szivek, and Hughes 1994).

Changing financial conditions, the reasoning of medical information that encourages supplier replacement, changing social standards, more intrusive government strategies, and changing socioeconomics present severe dangers to the power professional networks to participate in new associations with outside partners such as buyers, regulators, stakeholders, and substitutes (Begun and Lippincott 1993).

The SOP model resists that jurisdiction isn't settled

unequivocally. The S.A. model places that the profession must "consistently adjust to the changing universe of partners or stakeholders just as their changing and frequently conflicting standards" (Begun and Lippincott 1993).

A perfect representation of this is the directive of managed care to improve quality and, simultaneously, to abridge costs. By distinguishing more than 30 methodologies in five territories identifying with a fruitful variation. (Begun and Lippincott (1993) gives a sound structure to evaluate the level of experience professional achievement in their managing future.

Phase 1: Experiencing	Phase 2: (Re-) Constructing narrated experiences	Phase 3: Strategic decision making
• POS is experienced through interactions with and within the political context. • Trial and error	• Narrative are constructed based on experiencing • Time, plot and moral are	• Experience are used to inform and legitimize strategizing • Perceived POSs are reconsidered

falsifies assumptions about POS	attributed • Contextual threats and opportunities are identified	• Narrative itself is changed as it becomes appropriated

Table 4: Different phases of Model of the Strategic Adaptation

9.2. Redesign Model of workplace

This viewpoint, which we have named redesigning patient care (RPC), is firmly adjusted to Freidson's (1994) idea of a "bureaucratic labor market" and integrates a few heterogeneous ways to deal with rebuilding the medical services working environment and expert work. The methodology is grounded in the conviction that weakness is inherited in a hierarchical and inflexible work division. The allocation of the task is subjugated by licensure, certification, and legal jurisdiction. The RPC model perceives the opportunities for jurisdictional movements (as comprehensive in the SOP model) and how specialists appear to be willing to negotiate over probable future and design a casual division of work. Redesigned manifested function of the patient's care is to improve output and contain costs. Staffing patterns might be drastically changed by latent process and power in medical care and health care organizations.

The redesigning idea of the workforce of healthcare is not new. In the mid-1970s, the U.S. Department of Health, Education, and Welfare (DHEW) (1976) Report on Licensure and the American Hospital Associations. Ameriplan perceived that the training and licensure measures related to the medical division of work didn't give the adaptability expected to meet the changing medical services framework system. It was portrayed by "an inflexibility of design and capacity that isn't promptly versatile to quick change an undeniably apparent pattern in medical care."

The Licensure Report (U.S. Branch of Health and Human Services 1971) supported "tuning" the work division to address evolving issues. These reports drew intensely on crafted by Forgotson, Roemer, and Newman (1967). They contended that institutional licensure would give a system to planning new medical services callings and preparing programs while giving shields against "professional obsolescence" (Forgotson, Roemer, and Newman 1967).

During the 1990s, the RPC model has gotten related to quality improvement development and is stretched out to a broad scope of settings through various staff, both clinical and regulatory, who are trained to connect patient-based measures for improved clinical results and productivity. Courses at the Institute for Health Care Improvement, for instance, are joined by doctors, medical attendants, and clinical specialists who wish to build up the essential abilities to regard the expert working environment as an "object of inquiry."

It is stated by McLaughlin and Kaluzny (1990) that to the extent that TQM centers on errors of system, continuous improvement, aggregate duty, administrative initiative, responsibility, and interest. It is a type of executives drastically unique about traditional quality affirmation instruments related to emergency clinics and the callings. There is a developing agreement that multiskilled medical care representatives can broaden skilled jobs, lessening staff deficiencies, and decreasing expenses (Hyde and Fottler 1995).

Information systems design to catch bedside care and change information into an effective plan and result data, another base for updating patient consideration has been set up. Redesign nursing unit projects focus on care continuity, appropriate resources, professional growth, and patient satisfaction (Parsons and Murdaugh 1994).

It has been noted with great interest that the Agency for Health Care Policy and Research's Patient Outcome Research Team (PORT)' program imparts the health services researchers and other healthcare members like physicians how to identify the most effective medical procedures.

The said program has been started outside of the traditional medical and biomedical, and clinical research community, which is a most important department from conventional medical research and other development efforts, and it transcends RPC's partial view as restructuring nursing work and care. RPC's most important and expansive review an organized system in which both inpatient and ambulatory care will be streamlined to minimize and finish inefficiencies in this profession. The other RPC approach needs a helping strategy where different professions work to define how care is delivered or delivered.

9.3. The Consumer Sovereignty Model

While building on the long-held notion that healthcare in this nation is overwhelmingly a local event, Ezekiel Emanuel (1991) advocates a change in the healthcare system design around some small communities as small as 20,000 individuals who can change their vision of wanted healthcare services into prominent and significant plans and customized services in community health planning and research.

Along with the help of physicians, the care providers would search for equal or similar plans of their comfort level towards the covered benefits and their ethical ideals in a C.S. System. Albeit physicians will not be compelled to give up a plan given disagreements connected with the special and particular services, Emanuel (1991) especially recognizes that such situations may arise in which physicians' philosophy and plan hopes lie in fundamental conflict. As such, circumstances would compel a physician to seek alternative jobs (Emanuel 1991).

Emanuel's (1991) vision recognizes that:

(1) There is no globally recognized view of what makes an acceptable style of care and required or wanted benefits; and

(2) There seem some groups of such individuals who can collectively agree on the nature of the organization(s) to get the care and the range of services they hold as desirable.

The fears for the loss of medicine's neutralizing power under such a situation of consumer control are countered by Emanuel's (1991) proposals that, in the setting of medical and professional standards, standards defining the appropriateness of certain diagnostic tests and the most effective therapies for certain diseases, the community wouldn't be involved, by any means. On the contemporary, the "community might formulate alternate ethical policies by setting priorities among services, establishing guidelines for the treatment of incompetent patients, outlining the type of informed consent procedures to be instituted and the similar.

These areas later don't reject clinical decisions while guaranteeing doctor investment as "gatekeepers" of the local area's moral norms. Emanuel (1991) distinguishes Group Health

Cooperative of Puget Sound, which has a board cultivating local area considerations. One illustration of another association that utilizes solid shopper power standards, including city centers at the wellbeing community level.

At a full-scale level, the Oregon Health Decisions measure is an example of the health decision-making community. The management role under a C.S. model is to guarantee the designation of assets to meet community targets and enroll and hold a medical staff focused on the local area's vision of medical and health care.

Emanuel (1991) doesn't investigate the opportunities for decentralization in vertically coordinated systems and the organization of managed care. There is no motivation behind why a given system or HMO probably won't have a few communities with various visions for their maintenance. John Goodman (1995), leader of the National Center for Policy Analysis, offers help for the C.S. model in a conflict that while our present way to deal with customer strengthening through medical investment accounts is "somewhat crude and bureaucratic" (being founded on the objectives of HMOs). The future will be grounded on "people seeking after their circumstance in a serious commercial center." In this system, patients will positively significantly discover more about offering medical practice.

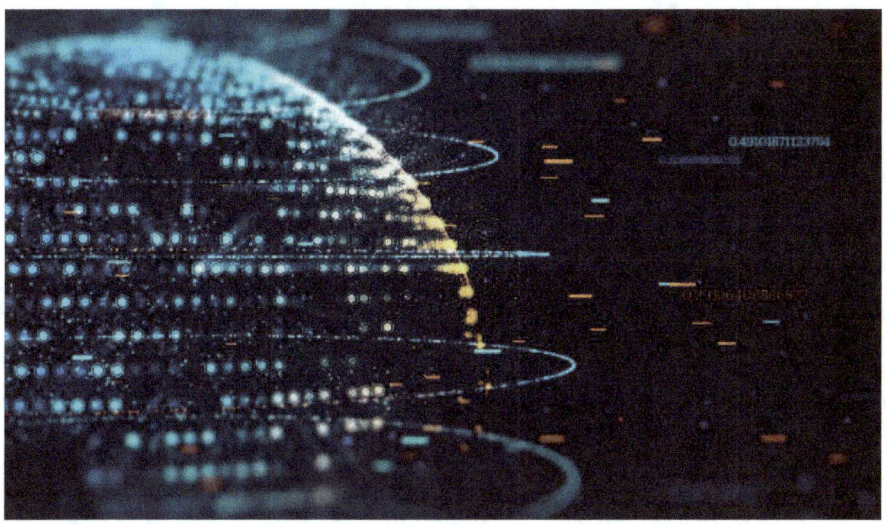

Innovation is always a great strategy in every field including healthcare too.

Chapter 10

Rule of

Healthcare Ethics

Regardless of whether your role is that of a doctor or a health care chairman, working in health care is both highly fulfilling and testing. Numerous operations and medicines have two benefits and drawbacks, and patients have their information and conditions to consider. The four standards of health care morals created by Tom Beauchamp and James Childress in the 1985 Principles of Biomedical Ethics give clinical professionals rules to settle on choices when they face muddled circumstances, including patients. The four standards of health care morals are autonomy, helpfulness, non-maleficence, and equity.

The fundamental meanings of every one of the four standards of health care morals are ordinarily known and utilized often in the English language. However, they take on exceptional importance when being used in a clinical setting. These standards assume a vital part in guaranteeing ideal patient wellbeing and care.

1. **Autonomy**: In medication, autonomy alludes to one side of the patient to hold command over their body. A health care professional can propose or exhort, yet any activities that endeavor to convince or pressure the patient into settling on a decision are an infringement of this guideline. Eventually, the patient should be permitted to settle on their own choices – regardless of whether the clinical supplier accepts these decisions are in that quiet's eventual benefits – autonomously and as per their qualities and convictions.

2. **Helpfulness**: This rule expresses that health care suppliers should do everything they can to profit the patient in every circumstance. All systems and medicines prescribed should be to do the most useful for the patient. To guarantee helpfulness, clinical experts should create and keep a high degree of expertise and information, ensure that they are prepared in the most current and best clinical practices, and think about their patients' conditions; what is useful for one tolerant won't important advantage another.

3. **Non-Maleficence**: Non-maleficence is most likely the most popular of the four standards. To put it plainly, it signifies "to do no damage." This rule is planned to be the ultimate objective for the entirety of a specialist's choices. It implies that clinical suppliers should consider whether others or society could be hurt by a choice made, regardless of whether it is made to support an individual patient.

4. **Justice**: The standard of equity expresses that there ought to be a component of decency on the whole clinical choices: reasonableness in choices that weight and advantage, just as an equivalent conveyance of scant assets and new therapies, and for clinical specialists to maintain relevant laws and enactment when settling on decisions.

10.1. Step by step instructions to maintain ethics in Healthcare management

Health care professionals now face fantastic troubles; all the while learning new monetary models, obliging the shopper market, and helping out external controls and organizations, interestingly puts enormous tension on care suppliers. This climate requires a restored center around morals. The models introduced by top management shows staff individuals how to perform morally. The choices that outcome from management's models decide an organization's moral culture. Considering this, health care chiefs notice the accompanying practices.

Ethical principle	Example of risk	Example of mitigation
Autonomy	• Patients can't exercise informed consent if they don't understand the risk and advantages of algorithms	• Ban black boxes: algorithms need to be made available for independent academic study.

Beneficence	- Healthcare AI models might emerge that primarily serve nonmedical functions such as targeted advertising.	- Prohibit sharing of personal health information with technology firms. Unless the downstream uses are explicitly for medical benefits.
Non-maleficence	- Massive data sets create potential for even de-identified health data sets to be used in ways that harms individuals.	- Implement short time limits on retention of health data by tech companies. Prohibit both sharing with third parties and re-identification.
Justice	- AI may exacerbate health disparities through exploitive pricing models.	- Develop reasonable pricing clauses and adapt intellectual property law to reflect ownership

			rights by public whose data were used to train the algorithms.

Table 5: Ethical principles of Healthcare with Examples

10.1.1 Arranging Organizational Ethics

The American College of Healthcare Executives (ACHE) distributes writing that assists directors with managing organizational morals. Strengthening Ethical Decision Making, the distribution fills in as a rule to help health care heads understand contemporary morals. The ACHE Ethics Toolkit traces how to settle on moral decisions and uncovers how organizations utilize the ACHE Code of Ethics in true applications. The affiliation likewise conveys the Ethical Policy Statements distribution, which health care managers use to make organizational rules. Chairpersons utilize the Ethics-Self Assessment Tool to design inner reviews and distinguish any shortcomings in organizational morals

10.1.2 Advancing Ethics in the Workplace

The National Association for Healthcare Quality (NAHQ) suggests an in-house health care quality professional manages moral culture. This expert oversees professional improvement preparing all through the organization and advances common friend backing and patient consideration in the caregiving setting.

Health care quality professionals advance corporate interest in community affiliations and gatherings and keep a conventional framework to address morals objections. NAHQ distributes the Code of Ethics for Healthcare Quality Professionals to guide subject matter experts and chairpersons.

10.1.3 Staff Member Ethics Education

Even though morals preparing has won in educational establishments for more than thirty years, the theme has gotten reestablished consideration, with various organizations framing to energize different critical interests to health care professionals. One essential worry among health care advocates includes morals preparing norms for explicit caregiver disciplines.

The Romanell Report suggests giving instruction credits (CME) to guarantee that health care professionals stay current with their morals preparing. The report also suggests utilizing theoretical devices, for example, role-playing and contextual analyses to give workers an unmistakable comprehension of how moral dynamic finds a way into the organizational culture.

Viable preparing programs help ingrain clinical morals and human qualities while advancing empathy toward patients, relatives, and different caregivers. Effectively keeping up continuous morals instruction requires a workforce who are focused on mentorship all through the organization.

10.1.4 Supporting Ethical Behavior

All organizations advance moral conduct through preparing or potentially writing. However, the everyday decisions made by organizational pioneers have more effect. Health care heads and directors can fill in as role models by tuning in to peers, tolerating ideas, and assuming liability for their activities. This commitment implies that upper management will get data with fair-mindedness.

Pioneers who don't transparently urge workers to shout out when untrustworthy occasions happen, ruining opportunities to improve their organization's personality. Health care chairpersons should characterize and demonstrate through model how much management esteems open revelations.

10.1.5 Sustaining Free Expression

Health care managers can eliminate the negative undertone and shame that typically accompanies whistle passing up re-outlining the demonstration... by introducing it as a high moral activity of making some noise or raising a worry. This point of view permits workers to see informant divulgences as typical and useful instead of if all else fails to inspire change. Moreover, managers can remind staff that patients are the essential worry inside the caregiving setting, underscoring caring reasoning for making some noise.

By causing staff individuals to have a sense of security to voice their interests, overseers construct a particular affinity that keeps little issues from transforming into significant issues. Morals disapproved of health care chairpersons comprehend that when representatives shout out, it's anything but an attack against the organization yet an opportunity to improve.

10.1.6 Debilitating Harassment

The health care field isn't insusceptible from work environment badgering. Over a portion of all ladies who work, regardless of the field or industry, report inappropriate behavior during their careers.

The Civil Rights Act of 1964 shields representatives from provocation because of sex, shading, or identity. In 1967, the Equal Opportunity Employment Committee (EEOC) corrected the demonstration to forestall age segregation.

These laws disallow managers and businesses from settling on wrong choices and expect bosses to find a way to forestall provocation. In any case, businesses can't address badgering claims except if staff individuals shout out when it happens. It is significant for workers to comprehend current provocation rights and announcing methodology unmistakably.

10.1.7 Keeping a Safe Work Environment

Health care chairpersons devise and ceaselessly keep up shields to secure representatives who raise work environment concerns. Administrators likewise request patients for criticism to recognize zones for development. This act of consistent criticism and improvement becomes progressively pertinent as new advancements keep driving the health care industry.

By noticing the acts of working environment morals, health care executives help create and advance model organizations. To keep up this culture, executives consistently review morals approaches. Notwithstanding, full organizational cooperation — from chiefs, managers, and all staff individuals — stays the main factor in maintaining a highly moral working environment culture.

Chapter 11

Importance of health care management motivation

H.R. (human resource) is fundamental to a successful healthcare system. From an economic perspective, the salaries of workers of health care share budgets of health in most countries. The gatekeeper of the health system is a health worker.

In the work environment, inspiration can be characterized as a "person's level of readiness to apply and keep an exertion towards goals of an organization." Motivation is firmly connected to work fulfillment, which holds laborers at their positions after some time (Vujicic, Marko, and Pascal, 2006).

The retention of healthcare workers decreases expenses to the health system's recruitment, employing, and situating new laborers and lessening vacant posts' probability.

As various countries presently experience a lack of qualified health workers, the deficiency of any healthcare specialist worker—particularly specialists and attendants—has serious consequences for individuals' wellbeing in that country.

The health care workers that are poorly motivated can harm the facilities of the individual and whole system. Unmotivated workers of health care fundamentally impact countryside areas. Health care workers regularly work longer hours, whose working environments have fewer assets than urban health care centers. They can generally feel isolated. Unmotivated healthcare workers are known to find employment elsewhere, either leaving the country and distant regions for work in bigger urban areas or relocating to different nations. Some disappointed health workers have been known to leave the medical field inside and out.

Inspiration is impacted by a set of social, proficient, and economic factors. There are numerous reasons health workers choose to remain at their jobs and remain motivated. Workers will be inspired and express occupation fulfillment if they believe they are viable at their positions and perform well. Healthy career development, adequate compensation, and working living conditions are the factors that contribute to job satisfaction and motivation.

Keeping a positive relationship with collaborators can increase inspiration. In an investigation in Ethiopia, attendants experienced more occupation fulfillment if they believed they had more meaningful self-governance to settle on their own choices concerning patient requirements.

Career development is the generally specializing possibility in a particular field or being advanced through workers positions. Specialists and workers working in countryside settings refer to restricted profession improvement openings as a demotivating factor. An investigation of South African specialist's doctors working in countryside areas found many complaints about not connecting to courses of online training to study specialty. Another problem is promotion lacking opportunity. It is reported that Tanzanian nurses worked ten years without a promotion. This has prompted terrible emotions, where the analysts call attention to that basic communication (Kotzee and Couper, 2006).

Having restricted proceeding with proficient advancement openings—or training during education or at work—is another significant subject among unhappy workers. In understaffed centers and emergency clinics in Tanzania, workers regularly perform assignments past their training extension. It can lead to demotivation and frustration.

Insufficient and obsolete medical resources and supplies at facilities and emergency clinics can contribute to health workers' frustration on the job. Workers contend that a shortage of sufficient assets disallows them from tackling their responsibilities. Specialists in South Africa revealed they left their work at provincial centers because of an absence of facilities, materials, and medical equipment.

Another issue is keeping a positive relationship with the board of management. For long periods, empty positions are left unfilled for expanding jobs for residual workers. Health care workers in rural areas usually complain absence of supervision from their directors or managers. Feedback from the staff is problematic. Manongi et al. state that negative feedback was received from their supervisors.

Objections about pay rates are another issue. Workers

in Uganda griped to analysts that they don't acquire sufficient compensation than other government employees of evenhanded callings. In Bangladesh, workers protested that they are not paid on time by the govt. Sometimes salary dispersal is usually behind six months.

Inspiration techniques should comprehensively move toward these mind-boggling issues: give freedoms to professional improvement, put forth attempts to guarantee sufficient pay, and advance positive workplaces, including ongoing oversight.

Realizing that there is room inside a health worker profession for additional improvement is a basic factor in propelling workers and permitting them to gather their networks' changing medical necessities. The expanding number of open positions, regardless of whether it is climbing the association progressive system or giving the capacity to learn new things. It is a fundamental marker of occupation fulfillment or job satisfaction. Career planning is institutional or personal that allows workers to increase job commitment. Health systems help workers with career planning. It can improve self-esteem and empower the maintenance of aspiring staff.

Salary increases may not be feasible in low-resource countries. Tino Maliselo and Rita Magawa suggest that providing more services and facilities (such as improved roads) in rural areas will be a more cost-effective way to boost motivation for health workers in those areas. Health workers in Asia and the Pacific esteem modern working environments with proper water and sanitation systems, as well as modern lighting and communication technology, according to a report.

This procedure can also be used by health care providers in other places. Providing better and more comfortable working environments increases the effectiveness and quality of service provided by health care staff. In Kenya, health facilities successfully improved staff morale and pride by implementing low-cost initiatives such as cleaning public areas, increasing flowers on-site, and providing free tea to employees in break rooms.

It's also crucial for health workers' motivation, efficiency, and decision to stay at work if they feel secure on the job. This involves concerns such as supplying clean water to health employees; ensuring that workers have sufficient supplies of protective equipment and are adequately qualified to handle chemicals; and making small changes to the physical environment – such as improving equipment ergonomics and reducing the amount of heavy lifting for health workers – reduces absenteeism.

It's also important to follow positive management guidelines and have quality supervision. This can be accomplished by enhancing the overall management efficiency. Employing professionally qualified managers with clear goals to spend more time with health staff, providing appropriate and positive input, and implementing consistent reward programs are only a few examples.

Deussom and Jaskiewicz suggest that well-designed performance-based funding schemes or other forms of payment-for-performance plans will strengthen accountability for specific services by requiring more or better oversight and verification. Staff would be more invested in achieving the facility's success targets if they are held more accountable.

However, difficulties do arise frequently. Quality control tools are often lacking among supervisors. Supervisors may have difficulty obtaining adequate transportation to visit health care providers. Managers often devote a significant amount of time to administrative tasks for donors and their administration.

It is not just the responsibility of their bosses to motivate health staff. Health care staff with a rural history or experience are more likely to choose to work in a rural environment. Policymakers and stakeholders at the national level also have a part to play. Evidence-based decision-making can be used to develop national policies to recruit, inspire, and retain health staff. This involves using valuable data to guide policy and decision-making. However, it can be difficult to know what to calculate when working with health systems, particularly in developing countries.

A cost-benefit analysis is needed for any incentive and retention strategy, since it allows policymakers to consider the benefits and drawbacks of particular initiatives. To ensure that proposed policy changes are thoroughly vetted, policymakers can bring together a diverse group of stakeholders. Finally, careful coordination is required to ensure that proper standards for health workers are established (Ditlopo et al., 2013).

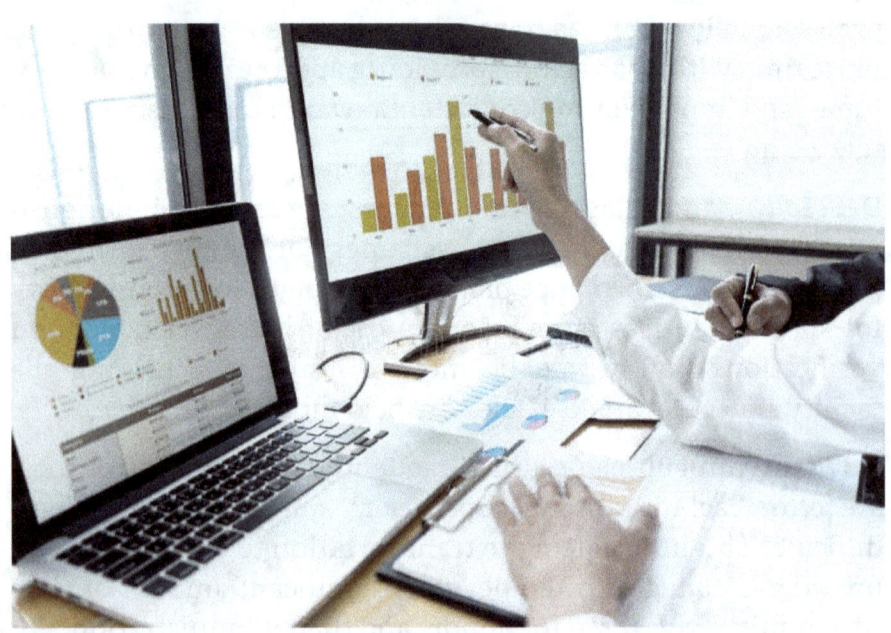

Chapter 12

Healthcare Strategic Planning

For the most part, the healthcare industry is too complicated and overwhelming for most people to comprehend. Because of technical advances or government orders, it is constantly evolving. It's becoming increasingly necessary to prepare for the healthcare organization's success. Your company will better prepare for the unexpected by planning for the future. A solid strategic plan benefits all levels of the business, no matter how big or small it is.

12.1. What is Healthcare Strategic Planning?

In healthcare organizations, strategic planning entails setting priorities and targets for where the company wants to go in the long run. You will make a strategy to accomplish these goals and objectives if you keep them in mind. You can't just set targets and objectives based on your own requirements. You must also adjust them to reflect current economic conditions, government policies, and technical advances.

In order for healthcare organizations to thrive, strategic planning is essential. Understanding how the company works is crucial to developing a successful business strategy for the entire healthcare system. You may need to examine the organization's hierarchy from time to time. Determining your company's priorities and charting a course to achieve them inspires your whole team to excel alongside you.

12.2. Why is Healthcare Strategic Planning Important?

12.2.1 Communication between all chains has improved

It's easy for departments at all levels to lose track of what's going on. Employees and customers alike want to make sure that the company has a long-term future. They want to know where the company is going and how you intend to get there. In healthcare management, effective preparation will help you build transparency and enhance communication. The main challenges, the organization's vision and priorities, and the measures to get there should all be addressed in your strategic plan. Your employees and stakeholders will have more trust and confidence in your business.

12.2.2 Creating and communicating a vision

With this in mind, you can have a positive effect at all levels of your business. Employees would be dedicated and encouraged to assist you in realizing your goals. Stakeholders will be able to make sound financial decisions with the courage and consistency they need. Strategic planning for healthcare facilities that is created, implemented, and shared will assist each of your employees in carrying out your vision for a prosperous future.

12.2.3 Employee motivation and commitment have increased.

Every one of your employees wishes to be seen and heard. Recognition by their superiors can have a significant effect on their success, commitment, and safety management. Every employee wishes to be given the authority to make decisions that will help the company. This also encourages them to go above and beyond the job description or performance evaluation's minimum reasonable criteria. Employees would be unmotivated to better themselves if their employer lacks a compelling goal and a well-executed game plan.

12.2.4 Authority and transformational leadership

Transformational leadership is a style of management that motivates workers to work harder and achieve greater results. It implements approaches that have been referenced in the literature on organizational behavior. Leaders who are transformational articulate their organization's mission, trust in their workers, and achieve high standards of success. It is important for strategic management to help your workers understand how their positions will contribute to your organization's mission and vision.

12.2.5 Collaboration and coordination among team members have improved.

In order to provide high-quality healthcare, team coordination and cooperation are necessary. Employees must collaborate in order for the company to succeed. The healthcare industry needs to work together to strengthen its efficiency and service. In the healthcare industry, effective strategic planning models will bring the staff together to provide high-quality care, excellent customer support, and improved productivity.

Before sharing your strategic plan with your staff, give it some thought. A well-thought-out and implemented strategic plan will help to enhance collaboration, performance accountability, and employee engagement. You will easily accomplish the organization's long-term goals if all levels work together in harmony.

Chapter 13

Marketing in the Healthcare Industry

Marketing concept Marketing is the investigation, planning, implementation, and control of meticulously organized programs aimed at achieving deliberate quality trades with target audiences in order to achieve organizational goals. It is heavily reliant on the organization's services being tailored to the needs and wants of the target market, as well as on the use of persuasive estimating, correspondences, and delivery to inform, convince, and service the business sectors. (Kotler and Roberta N. Clarke, Kotler and Clarke, Roberta N. Clarke, Roberta N. Clarke (1987)

13.1. Marketing Healthcare Services is a concept that has been around for a long time.

Marketing healthcare services entails making healthcare or Medicare services available to different customer groups in such a way that they receive high-quality services at a reasonable cost, at the right time and place, and in a professional manner.

13.2. Significant marketing challenges exist for healthcare providers.

Meyer and Franc (2011) emphasized that marketing has come a long way since its broad introduction into healthcare in the 1980s. It has, however, seen both good and poor times along the way. Despite the fact that many hospitals hired senior marketing executives and began to integrate marketing philosophy and practice into their operations, it was never widely adopted or accepted for a variety of reasons, including the following:

• Many senior leaders believed they understood the concepts, but they never assigned the organizational, operational, or financial responsibility for putting the concepts into action.

• Marketing did not always translate well from traditional item and service promotion (with its emphasis on publicizing and deals) to health-care services promotion.

• Healthcare marketing was not well understood or defined.

• When marketing was implemented in hospitals, all accounts were rehearsed at incredible levels within the organisation. It was often distorted as selling or publicizing, or thought to be inseparable from traditional advertising, raising money, or advancement, which cheapened its far-reaching use and extreme usefulness to the organisation. However, division-level supervisor inclusion was often restricted, which exacerbated the problem.

In the healthcare sector, there are a variety of marketing concepts to consider.

13.3. Definition of production

According to Kotler (2013), one of the most well-established market ideas is that consumers will gravitate toward products that are generally available and modest. Here, management is focused on achieving high creation efficiency, low costs, and widespread distribution. Meyer and Franc (2011) have stated that it is not about providing low-cost, widely available health care; rather, reliable and efficient services are provided.

13.4. The definition of the product

Shoppers choose product concept compositions with the highest consistency, execution, or artistic highlights. Managers of these companies are focused on creating quality products and developing them over time. They believe that a superior mousetrap can lead people to the most efficient routes to their doors. Before the 1980s, the notion of marketing in the healthcare industry was misunderstood and there was a belief that only the disabled required a doctor and should seek out a physician. This discernment has become an infection in the health-care industry that has slowed its growth.

13.5. The definition of sale

The selling principle, according to Keller (2013), states that if customers and companies are left alone, they will not purchase enough of the organization's goods. As a result, the company must make a concerted effort to market and promote its products. The sale term is most vigorously used for unsought products, such as insurance, health papers/articles, encyclopedias, and funeral plots, according to Kotler and Keller. In the health-care sector, products such as health insurance are available. Low-income people clarified to Ahuja (2004) that insurance was never considered an option in the past. They were believed to be unable to save and pay the premium because they were bad. As a result, the government accepted responsibility for fulfilling the poor's health-care needs.

13.6. The marketing strategy

Marketing principles originated in the mid-1950s, according to Philip Kotler (2013), when companies moved to a customer-centered, feel and reply philosophy. In 1960, Harvard Professor Levitt emphasized that the marketing philosophy is centered on the needs of customers, specifically the idea of meeting the needs of the consumer using the product and the whole cluster of items associated with making, delivering, and eventually consuming it. In their book, Meyer and Franc (2011) stated that senior health executives should not be complacent when it comes to marketing because it is the organization's voice.

13.7. The principle of holistic marketing

Beyond conventional marketing principles, today's best marketers understand the need for a more comprehensive, coherent strategy. When it comes to marketing, holistic marketing recognizes that everything matters, and that a deep, integrated perspective is often required. Relationship marketing, integrated marketing, internal marketing, and success marketing are all elements of comprehensive marketing (Keller and Philip Kotler, 2013).

13.8. As a rule, healthcare marketing

Hospital marketing, according to Ashok Anantram (2009), President of Business Growth at Apollo Hospitals in Chennai, is the same in the product and service industries. Interaction between producers and customers in marketing. Healthcare marketing is a difficult equation to solve since, in most cases, the manufacturer, the doctor, is also the marketer because production and consumption happen at the same time. Patients are the best ambassadors, so it's important to think about their needs and have the best treatment possible. Their fears must be resolved in order for them to return to the same facility.

13.9. The significance of health product marketing

According to Leonard Berry (1999), professor of marketing at the Lowry Mays College and Graduate School of Business, the most important customer service is health care because we are directly influenced by it every day. People shape opinions about local hospitals based on stories from friends, relatives, and coworkers, according to Shelly (2013). She goes on to say that current patients are an effective and useful marketing tool for the hospital. As a result, marketing aids in the maintenance of good relationships with current customers, who play an important role in referring friends and family to the hospital, thus increasing sales.

13.10. Effects of Marketing on Healthcare system

The unique advancement of life has unavoidably influenced the healthcare frameworks creating critical changes and forcing healthcare marketing as a fundamental component of health brands. Healthcare is a field in perpetual advancement, the plenty of opportunities animating inventiveness, excitement, and will abuse the experts in the field.

As the way of thinking and marketing strategies in different fields can't discover appropriateness in the healthcare services, healthcare needs their methodology and present certain highlights that are not found in different ventures.

Healthcare marketing is an interdisciplinary field through its explicitness since it utilizes certain ideas, strategies, and methods explicit both to traditional and social marketing. The particularity of healthcare marketing is that there are services and markets yet no cash same. This implies the viability of its application can be found in the picture of a healthy populace, the discovery of a persistently sick class of individuals, guaranteeing the therapy of sick individuals by experiencing the full restoration measure, professional reintegration, social reintegration of sick individuals, and so on The utilization of marketing in the field of healthcare was forced by the issues in the health of the general public.

An effective marketing approach includes inside and out examination of the patients' requirements, distinguishing idle necessities, and offering new health services that patients have not expressly mentioned.

Patients' contribution in accomplishing the clinical demonstration has become a need of present existence with wide and complex implications, not just past changing the mindset of the suppliers yet also with critical changes like way of life, utilization propensities, and medicine of recipients. As the day-by-day measure advances, change will be major to our reality's central motivation: life. Moreover, this will, without a doubt, bear the impediment of how the relationship will orchestrate the requirement for health. Primary changes power health frameworks to quicken towards the future, thinking about the current requirements, and the future procedure can't be practical without performing management and marketing capacities.

The marketing of healthcare services contrasts basically through the idea of interest for health services. Also, the recipient may not be the marketing effort's objective, the physician being the person who chooses what, where, when, and how much will be accommodated a specific service. The chief might be the specialist, the health plan agent, a relative. Healthcare services likewise vary where the item can be extremely mind-boggling and may not be handily conceptualized. Many of the healthcare systems, particularly those dependent on innovation, are convoluted and hard to disclose to an individual who hasn't had some expertise in that specific field.

Another healthcare challenge, particularly for service suppliers, is that not all potential customers are considered alluring for a specific service. While service suppliers are needed to offer types of assistance to all candidates, paying little mind to their capacity to pay, there are certain classifications of patients whom the advertiser may not urge to demand a specific service. The advertiser faces the test of drawing in clients to healthcare organizations, nonetheless, without pulling in an excessive number of from the class of the individuals who are probably going to address monetary obligations.

Over the previous decade, healthcare has encountered many marketing patterns that have generally adjusted marketing. These patterns are the follows:

- From a mass marketing way to deal with a more explicit methodology.
- From picture marketing to service marketing.
- From "one measure for all" to personalization.
- From the accentuation on a health scene to a dependable relationship.
- From "disregarding" the market to showcase insight.
- From low-tech to high-tech

Marketing assumes a significant part in encouraging healthcare professionals to make, convey, and offer some benefit to their objective market. Current advertisers start from clients instead of from items or services. They are keener on building a feasible relationship than on guaranteeing a solitary exchange. Their point is to make a high degree of purchaser fulfillment to get back to a similar provider. Advertisers have utilized numerous conventional strategies that incorporate marketing research, item plan, dispersion, evaluating, publicizing, limited-time deals, and deals management. These techniques should be joined by new ones, identified with innovation and new ideas, to pull in clients through messages and offers.

Albeit the customer ordinarily gets the vast majority of the data about an item through the business media. The primary data comes from suggestions or freely accessible autonomous specialists. The two classifications of sources give correlative capacities; business media – advises, while individual or master sources legitimize or potentiate the assessment cycle. For instance, physicians often get some answers concerning new medications from business sources. However, they go to different physicians for real sentiments.

Albeit much has been expounded on subconscious choices, current models take a gander at the cycle from a psychological point of view, which implies the purchaser/patient, makes his own decisions on a factual premise.

While trying to address an issue, the patient expects certain advantages from the picked health service and supplier. The patients' perspectives, decisions, and inclinations about specific brands through a strategy of assessing these brands' credits build up an allowance of faith-based expectations about the ascribes that compare to each brand.

The fundamental entertainer who denotes the interaction of creation and conveyance of healthcare services is the patient, and his quality is essential for the conveyance framework.

In the field of healthcare services, the presentation happens just within sight of the healthcare buyer and his wiliness to the service. Subsequently, the shopper turns into a key factor for any service; the buyer connects with the provider and becomes a co-supplier of the service, taking an interest in time and exertion in the conveyance interaction.

Healthcare shoppers are effectively or latently engaged with the conveyance. However, their quality has suggestions for the clinical organization's action because any expert who meets the patient will add to the service creation. Moreover, any specific component, which the healthcare customer meets, is important for the health service conveyance measure; truth be told, any progressions happening at the spot of service conveyance will prompt changes in the patient's conduct.

From a marketing point of view, the way toward giving healthcare services should be led in full consistence with patient necessities, exercises are being intended to meet these prerequisites. Notwithstanding, accomplishing such an objective infers the ID of all places of obstruction of healthcare staff with the healthcare service buyers and the appraisal of the degree to which the exercises completed at these focuses compare to the patients' necessities and assumptions. Since the health services customer's conduct is hard to foresee, the presence of the patient in the conveyance cycle might be a wellspring of significant vulnerability.

A long way from having uninvolved conduct, the purchaser has different capacities to create services as a co-maker, which decides numerous experts to think of him as an outside human asset.

Patient satisfaction should be the primary target of any healthcare organization, and this requires exhaustive information on their necessities and assumptions. Giving a high-quality healthcare service depends on gathering certain prerequisites with the goal that the service achieves the level wanted by the patient. To acquire the trust of healthcare shoppers, the specific staff of the organizations in the field should be more open to the desires, ideas, patient grievances and, simultaneously, become more delicate to their interests. This methodology's viability relies upon how the clinical organization has a powerful correspondence with patients, presents the right picture of the health service, conveys the guaranteed service appropriately, and presents a perpetual worry for the service's persistent improvement of the assumptions for the patients.

By acting in a dynamic and unusual climate, (to endure), the health service supplier should have the option to identify the opportunities and dangers of the market on which it works. In this unique circumstance, the detailing of a reasonable, sound, and express procedure by the clinical unit is critical in expecting its future and critical vulnerability in action.

The marketing methodology is how an organization acts affected by ecological elements. In pragmatic terms, marketing methodologies diagram away following the investigation of natural elements. The marketing strategy characterizes its overall activity system to do its whole movement, including a few methodologies.

Building up the marketing arrangements and methodologies explicit to health services giving units is a perplexing interaction. Considering numerous interior and outside factors, the interdependencies and molding join between them, just as the great or ominous effect they can apply on the health unit, they should be dissected inside and out, interrelated, and deciphered for settling on vital and firm choices concerning the future improvement of the clinical establishment.

The nature of services addresses the center of the marketing procedure in the field of health services. Fruitful organizations in the healthcare field have a reasonable, serious procedure that enables and compels them to adjust to ecological conditions. The healthcare services field's marketing system is the clinical organization's demeanor corresponding to the marketing climate and, simultaneously, its situation according to its segments.

Patients have countless such alternatives regarding the decision of healthcare services and suppliers that the lone way the healthcare practices can truly be recognized is by building up an all-around separated, important, and exceptional proposition close by a marketing methodology adjusted to the advanced period.

A significant proposition should have the accompanying qualities:

- It is valid
- The worth offered is better than the one of the opposition
- It is imperative to the objective public
- It is paramount and simple to recall
- It is hard to duplicate by the opposition.

As indicated by a Harvard Business Review, 64% of the customers have "veritable basic qualities" as the real effect on their relationship with the brand.

Today, significant healthcare organizations center on substance to dominate the race of advanced matchless quality. Content marketing techniques for the healthcare field are not just about writing for a blog and delivering specific outcomes. Since hospitals are connected to patients and physicians, advanced marketing is the best approach to carry this cycle to a new level.

As of now, the advanced substance helps assemble positive brand impressions. The utilization of new advanced marketing methodologies is fundamental to amplify marketing costs' proficiency and create higher bring rates back. By applying inventive health marketing standards to revitalize the clinical organization's marketing activities, organizations will want to all the more likely position their service offers to customers.

For healthcare suppliers, the utilization of educational websites or articles distributed via web-based media can be powerful approaches to remain pertinent to patients. Besides, implanting focused watchwords into the substance can add marketing support.

For organizational marketing to be viable, the computerized stages in which the organization will work should be recognized, the objective public should be divided accurately, and tweaked marketing messages should reverberate with the crowd.

To comprehend the effect of marketing systems on the nature of healthcare services, it is critical to see the present clinical buyer who likes to search for clinical data on the web, where he likewise has an abundance of healthcare services, healthcare suppliers, audits from patients who reached the supplier, and so forth

With computerized marketing, nearly everything can be followed and estimated. Healthcare professionals and healthcare organizations don't have to know what works and what doesn't work. With the assistance of marketing execution data, healthcare professionals and healthcare organizations can settle on an educated choice on the best way to improve their endeavors, alongside the capacity to consistently quantify and assess them.

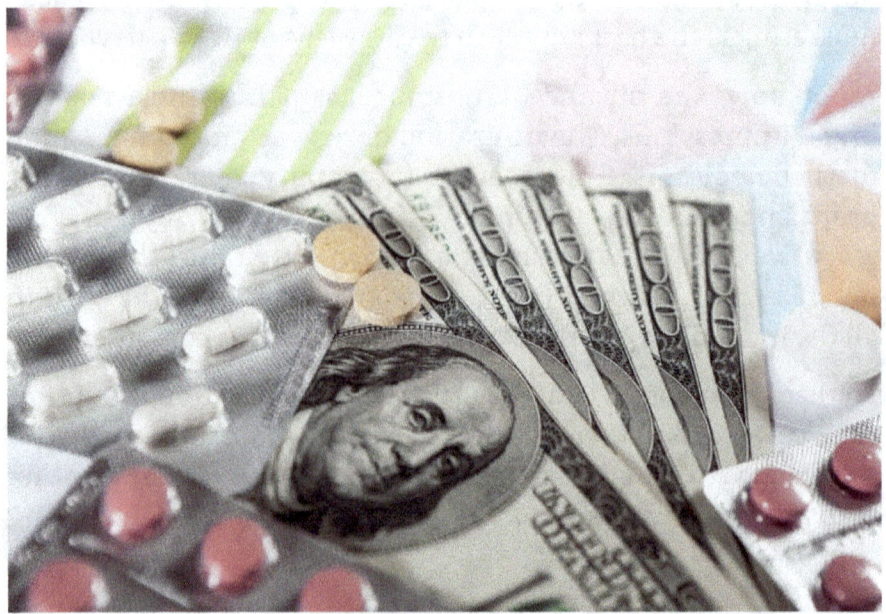

The healthcare business can fundamentally expand its inclusion and adequately draw in buyers with advanced marketing strategies.

As the marketing progress develops, organizations are moving towards more advanced ways to deal with buyers' stay. Advanced marketing costs have been the highest ever, with healthcare organizations spending more than $ 2.5 billion on marketing, assessed at $ 4 billion by 2020.

In this unique circumstance, 44% of the marketing costs for health-related items and services are devoted to portable and computerized stages. Television promoting costs have dropped to under 33% and are relied upon to keep on diminishing. The expense adequacy of setting an item or service on TV appears to, at this point don't legitimize the venture.

How customers utilize the web to discover hospital units and healthcare supplier's advances for shrewd gadgets. With over 80% of the patients who now and again use cell phones to either distinguish or communicate with physicians, it is fundamental to reconfigure marketing activities to fit the time we live in more readily. Likewise, as Google reconfigures its inquiry calculations to support versatile cordial sites, presently, it is the perfect chance to focus on reconsidering computerized promotions.

Simultaneously, the marketing blend system is fundamental in clinical organizations to guarantee their prosperity. Along these lines, the system prompts a huge effect on the clinical organization, including its presentation estimated by tolerant satisfaction, the co-appointment of arranged marketing endeavors to address organizational execution being fundamental.

Like this, the advantages of actualizing marketing procedures are

- to improve the upper hand,
- to build the permeability,
- to make a strong standing among patients,
- to comprehend the necessities and assumptions for shoppers,
- to comprehend the patients' view of the quality and aftereffects of their experience inside the clinical organization, offering important encounters to patients and building a solid, compelling, predominant brand on the health services market.

Chapter 14

Healthcare

Profession

Healthcare associations have many clinical, administrative, and uphold experts to convey health care service to their patients. The Bureau of Labor Statistics (BLS) demonstrated nearly 16 million positions in hospitals, workplaces of wellbeing experts, nursing and private care offices, home medical care administrations, and outpatient settings (Torpey, 2014).

The biggest business setting in medical services in hospitals and the biggest classification of medical services laborers is enlisted attendants, with 2.7 million positions, 61% of which are in emergency clinics (BLS, 2014h). As per the BLS, 691,400 doctors and specialists held positions in 2012 (BLS, 2014e).

Progressively, doctors are deciding to practice in huge gatherings or be utilized by emergency clinics instead of in performance or little practices. In 2013, Jackson Healthcare re-directed an overview of doctors and discovered 26% were hired by hospitals, an increment of 6% over the earlier year. Ownership stakes in rehearses, solo practices, and self-employed entity situations declined in a similar period (Vaidya, 2013).

Employment offers doctors a place of refuge in an unpredictable medical care climate. Under the umbrella of a clinic or other huge health care association, they have better work hours, advantages, and downtime, which they couldn't generally bear in little or solo practice. Normally, the extent of hire doctors will keep on filling in the coming decade. In 2012, doctor partners held 86,700 positions, more than 55% of which were in wandering medical care administrations, including doctor rehearses, about 20% were in clinics, and the rest in nursing care offices and government settings (BLS, 2014f).

Allied health experts comprise an expansive cluster of 28 health science experts, including, yet not restricted to, anesthesiologist associates, clinical colleagues, respiratory specialists, and surgical technologists (Commission on Accreditation of Allied Health Education Programs, 2015). As a health care manager, these measurements imply that in numerous cases, you will be working with a blend of individuals with one or the other pretty much schooling than you have. It additionally implies you won't have the clinical abilities that these medical care suppliers have—a scary situation, most definitely.

Rather than clinical skill, you will bring a foundation that empowers you to improve the climate in which these exceptionally individual staffs convey medical care services. You will be the individual liable for ensuring medical nurses, specialists, and other medical care experts have the assets to give protected and effective patient care. Your job will be to give and screen the foundation and cycles to make the health care association receptive to the patients and the representatives' requirements. The more you comprehend clinical medical care experts, the more ready you will be to take care of your work as a health care administrator.

14.1. Allied health

Allied health experts are engaged in a wide range of healthcare services that give clinical and populace care. The Association of Schools of Allied Health Professions (ASAHP) includes numerous projects inside its affiliated organizations, including athletic preparing, dietetics, occupational therapy, physical therapy, and respiratory treatment. There are just about 200 perceived allied health careers. Two careers alluded to on occasion as allied health career, nursing and doctor assistants, give a significant and different exhibit of essential care and preventive administrations.

14.1.1 Schooling/Training

Allied health students are prepared to get procedural abilities and to assess, analyze, and possibly treat ailments. Instructive educational plans remember guidance for research, result estimations, and quality of care issues. These are largely focal ideas in populace wellbeing. Prevention and health advancement correspondence procedures likewise are educated to professionals for use during single client advising meetings.

14.1.2 Clinical Prevention and Population Health Services

Allied health experts regularly engage, either autonomously or as a medical care group component, in the continuous assessment and evaluation of patients' wellbeing needs. Albeit a small segment of allied health, experts work exclusively in the public well-being field, most work as a clinical medical care group component. Notwithstanding the specific position they hold, these people should work inter expertly inside the medical care framework.

For instance, diabetes training programs for patients generally depend on the hard work of nurses and dieticians who work cooperatively with patients and different clinicians to accomplish healthy, effective results.

14.1.3 Difficulties/Future Opportunities

Most ASAHP schooling programs incorporate clinical prevention and populace wellbeing educational plans in their courses. Notwithstanding, the focal point of the vast majority of these subjects stays on clinical care. The ASAHP finished an investigation to survey whether its allied health universities utilized the Clinical Prevention and Population Health Curriculum Framework in required curricula. Although study respondents announced that their courses showed counteraction and wellbeing advancement ideas, preventive medication was a necessary subject in just the accompanying projects: athletic preparing (60%); dental sciences (64%); nursing (78%); doctor aides (100%); and respiratory treatment (75%). The Curriculum Framework should be unequivocally elevated to incorporate well-being advancement and disease prevention training in allied health schools (Jackson, 2010).

14.2. Dentistry

Dentistry, as defined by the American Dental Association House of Delegates, is The assessment, diagnosis, prevention, and additionally treatment (nonsurgical, surgical, or related methodology) of illnesses, disorders as well as states of the oral cavity, maxillofacial region, and additionally the adjacent and related structures and their effect on the human body; given by a dental specialist inside the extent of his/her schooling, preparing and experience, and as per the morals of the career and relevant law.

14.2.1 Education/Training

The Competencies for the New General Dentist, received by the American Dental Education Association House of Delegates, features the significant job of wellbeing advancement inside the field of dentistry. It expresses that overall dental specialists should be skillful at giving prevention, mediation, and instructive procedures; take part with dental and other medical care experts in understanding administration and wellbeing advancement, and add to the improvement of oral health past those served in conventional practice settings.

14.2.2 Clinical Prevention and Population Health Services

The major clinical preventive administrations gave by dental experts presently center around hazard evaluation for illnesses of the periodontium, the administration of dental caries by hazard assessment, and the early discovery of oral malignant growth. Albeit most of these administrations are individual clinical administrations, they give a chance to health education and advancement that reaches out into local area-based administrations. Dental specialists are very much situated to give proficient exhortation and take public approach promotion jobs, for example, those taken during water fluoridation endeavors to improve the populace's oral wellbeing. With an end goal to improve wellbeing advancement and populace wellbeing, dental experts team up with other medical care suppliers in proficient preparing programs. For instance, dental experts instruct students in clinical, nursing, and doctor assistants training programs.

14.2.3 Challenges/Future Opportunities

Expanding the clinical interactions among dental and other wellbeing experts could improve wellbeing results. For instance, the prevention, recognition, and treatment of conditions, for example, poor oral hygiene in the old populace, could be improved with a more joint effort. Strategies to build cooperation among medical services experts in the clinical setting are required. Furthermore, while the arrangement of oral health schooling and counteraction guidance is a significant errand of dental experts, repayment for advising time is insufficient. During the following quite a few years, expanded interest for admittance to dental consideration is likely. Authorizing changes are expected to allow the free act of dental hygienists and midlevel specialists in school-based dental projects, preschool youngster care focuses, nursing homes, and private settings, for example, detainment centers and homeless offices (American Dental Association, n.d).

14.3. Nursing

Nursing is the biggest healthcare career, with an expected 3.0 million registered nurses (RNs) in the U.S. as per the 2008 National Sample Survey of Registered Nurses. The specific obligations of individual nurses are reliant on the job, work on setting, populace served, and claim to a special area of the medical care practice they are hired. All nurses are set up to survey a patient's wellbeing, give clinical treatment, and teach patients and families.

14.3.1 Education/Training

Clinical prevention and populace health are fundamental curricular parts in the broadly perceived educational plan rules for baccalaureate, master's, and specialist of nursing practice programs. The curricular norms are needed by the public nursing authorizing body for baccalaureate and graduate nursing programs, the Commission of Collegiate Nursing Education. All baccalaureate-arranged medical attendants have required coursework and clinical encounters in the local area and public health. Also, a few nurses decide to practice at the alumni level in public health.

14.3.2 Clinical Prevention and Population Health Services

Clinical prevention and populace health is an important segment of most nursing practice. Nursing services incorporate health hazard assessments; usage of danger decreases procedures for people and networks; health training and advising for patients, families, and gatherings; controlling strategies of chronic diseases, and helping patients and families decipher and survey health data utilization of advancements.

Educated nurses at the graduate education level give a great part of the country's essential care and chronic disease management administrations. They achieve this in an assortment of settings, including local area or public health centers, private or gathering practice offices, clinics, long haul care and restoration services, and acute care services. Nurses who have graduate-level public health preparation give administration in arranging and executing general wellbeing projects and activities at the local, state, and public levels.

Notwithstanding their field of training, nurses are basic individuals from bury proficient groups and extensively affect health results when their extent of training is amplified. A survey of magnet medical clinics found that nurse's contribution in dynamic cycles corresponded with improved patient results.

14.3.3 Challenges/Future Opportunities

Perhaps the best zone of nursing commitment is in essential care practice and chronic ailment management. Repayment for administrations in those regions is deficient, be that as it may, and needs improvement. Advanced Practice Registered Nurses (APRNs), especially nurse practitioners (NPs) and certified nurse-midwives (CNMs), could make a more significant commitment to meeting the country's essential care needs. Be that as it may, many state guidelines limit the extent of APRNs' training (e.g., restricted prescriptive power, required doctor oversight, and no quick charging for administrations). Authorizing and administrative changes are expected to permit APRNs to rehearse all the more freely and their full extent of arrangement (Commission on, n.d).

14.4. Pharmacy

Pharmacists are the medicine use specialists or drug experts in the healthcare framework. They give medication treatment management, organize frameworks of medicine distribution and administering, interface with patients and prescribers, and participate in the arrangement of clinical and local area-based preventive administrations.

14.4.1 Education/Training

The Accreditation Council for Pharmacy Education is the certifying office for professional degree programs prompting the Pharmacy Doctor. In 2007, the accreditation norms were reconsidered to necessitate that pharmacy graduates be equipped to "advance health improvement, wellbeing, and infection counteraction in collaboration with patients, networks, in danger populaces, and different individuals from an interprofessional group of medical services suppliers." The drug specialist's training incorporates conduct change systems, such as persuasive talking, raising patient mindfulness and instruction, and adjusting practices that affect well-being. In 2009, 97.1% of graduating students from 83 universities and schools of pharmacy concurred or firmly concurred that the PharmD program at their particular establishments set them up to advance health and sickness prevention administrations.

14.4.2 Clinical Prevention and Population Health Services

The arrangement of patient care administrations for the ideal utilization of prescriptions at the individual and populace levels, the efficient and viable administration of the medicine dissemination and use frameworks, and the advancement of health and infection avoidance structure the establishment of the job of pharmacists practically speaking. As promptly available local area suppliers, pharmacists are very much situated to convey avoidance messages that are reliable with those of different individuals from an inter-professional health care group. Pharmacists often give clinical prevention and populace health administrations that incorporate immunizations, smoking-discontinuance programs, nutrition help, family planning schooling, epidemiologic surveillance, improvement of wellbeing proficiency, and anti-microbial administration. Pharmacists are perceived as vital to improving patient well-being results, particularly for those with ongoing ailments who benefit from prescription treatment and group-based ways to deal with care. For instance, drug specialists can assist patients with diabetes, managing complex medication regimens, and meet glycemic control objectives. This community pharmacy diabetes board program has been appeared to decrease medical care costs and improve patient satisfaction.

14.4.3 Challenges/Future Opportunities

The Health Resources and Services Administration perceives the significance of the pharmacist joining sites that serve needy or underserved populaces and supports this incorporation through the Patient Safety and Clinical Pharmacy Collaborative. Although private guarantor inclusion is expanding, scholarly pharmacy sponsors these administrations' arrangements, and more prominent financial pay are required. What's more, extending freedoms to reimburse pharmacists for inclusion in sickness the executives would be beneficial. Academic and expert drug store associations are focused on expanding patient admittance to clinical counteraction and populace wellbeing services. Access to drug specialists gave clinical avoidance, and populace wellbeing administrations are accessible. Prodded by incorporating prescription treatment the board for focused people in Medicare Part D, an increasing number of third-party payers, including some state Medicaid programs and self-insured managers, are adding admittance to drug specialist gave care as a covered benefit. Patients will have expanded admittance to prescription treatment the executive's administrations across the medical services continuum as arrangements of the Patient Protection and Affordable Care Act expected on improving consideration coordination, and quality is actualized (Accreditation Council for Pharmacy Education, n.d).

14.5 Physicians

Physicians are Doctors of Medicine (MDs) or Doctors of Osteopathic Medicine (DOs). They are authorized to endorse meds and give clinical therapy and administrations in any medical specialty, going from psychiatry to medical procedures. Osteopathic clinical schools give additional preparation on all-encompassing consideration, the musculoskeletal situation, and osteopathic manipulative treatment. Doctors work in an assortment of settings that incorporate medical clinics, outpatient centers; educational foundations; health divisions; legislative offices; and nongovernmental associations, such as promotion gatherings, drug organizations, and insurance agencies.

14.5.1 Education/Training

Physician training includes prevention and populace wellbeing in medical school and residency preparation. The Liaison Committee on Medical Education, the certifying expert for MD-granting schools, and the American Osteopathic Association Commission on Osteopathic College Accreditation certifies osteopathic medication universities. Both remember preventive medication and public health for their educational plan principles. Residency training likewise incorporates public health standards and abilities. A few doctors decide to have practical experience in preventive medicine and public health and become Preventive Medicine doctors. Preventive Medicine residency programs train doctors on the accompanying center abilities: biostatistics; the study of disease transmission; ecological and occupational health; arranging, organization, and assessment of wellbeing administrations; and the act of avoidance in clinical medication, wellbeing strategy, and management.

14.5.2 Clinical Prevention and Population Health Services

Physician practice clinical prevention and populace health in an assortment of jobs and settings. Essential consideration doctors center on sickness prevention and health advancement, giving preventive screening administrations and health advising to their patients. Moreover, as expressed in a 2007 IOM report, Training Physicians for Public Health Careers, most doctors also partake in public health exercises, even though they would not distinguish themselves as public health physicians. For instance, a physician who recognizes and treats an outbreak of influenza in a community health clinic is rehearsing public health. Truly, physicians were pioneers in public health. Albeit the public health labor force is more assorted now, doctors who work in general wellbeing still frequently expect such influential positions as overseer of constant sickness anticipation and wellbeing advancement program at a neighborhood wellbeing office, head of a state wellbeing office, or as a senior public wellbeing executive at a legislative office or nongovernmental association.

Physicians work in groups with other healthcare experts in different sorts of training settings. As expressed before, physicians are regularly in administrative roles inside the group and depend on all colleagues to work durably to care.

14.5.3 Challenges/Future Opportunities

Like the other health professions, repayment for clinical time spent on preventive health counseling and screening needs improvement. Another likely territory of improvement is to build openings for inter-professional preparation. As expressed in the 2003 IOM report A Bridge to Quality, "Health experts are approached to work in interdisciplinary groups, frequently to help those with constant conditions, yet they are not instructed together or prepared in group-based abilities." Increasing inter-professional instruction and preparing in clinical school, residency, and practical settings is advisable.

Numerous medical students report that they need fitting preparation in public health and populace health points. Maximizing efforts to address this deficiency is additionally suggested. Patients and networks may benefit if doctors had a superior comprehension of the public health framework and the chances to add to improving populace wellbeing. Master boards have suggested that anticipation and public health content in clinical training should be improved and have identified the substance regions they felt would generally apply to doctors. Furthermore, an extension of the quantity of DO–MPH and MD–MPH programs and expanded subsidizing for Preventive Medicine residency projects would build doctors' chances to participate in populace health training and ensuing practice (National Academies Press, n.d).

14.6. Physician Assistants

Physician assistants (PAs) are authorized healthcare professionals who practice medicine with doctor oversight. PAs perform actual assessments, analyze and treat diseases, arrange and decipher symptomatic tests, give preventive health guiding and services, aid a medical procedure, and recommend meds and clinical gadgets. PAs, rehearsing inside a doctor PA group model, practice self-rule in a clinical dynamic and offer a wide cluster of indicative and remedial services. Physician administrators delegate the obligation to the PAs with whom they work through the extent of training rules, which may develop as the doctor partners get new abilities while in clinical practice.

14.6.1 Education/Training

Physician assistants are one of a kind in that most are prepared for essential care. The generalist model often used to prepare PAs can be supplemented likewise by preparing careful and subspecialty care. Most preparing programs prepare their alumni to follow general rules and best practices for health advancement and illness anticipation, for example, those suggested by the U.S. Preventive Services Task Force and CDC. Numerous PAs also prepare inspirational talking and social modification methods, which help patients adhere to healthy lifestyles.

14.6.2 Clinical Prevention and Population Health Services

Physician assistants can convey a wide scope of infection counteraction and health advancement services like other essential care suppliers. These services incorporate patient training and advising about healthy ways of life and shirking of practices known to influence a patient's health or personal satisfaction contrarily. A 2008 enumeration report from the American Academy of Physician Assistants uncovered that over 43% of PAs worked in bunch practices or solo physician offices, and more than 33% were working in hospitals. The excess PAs were situated in-country facilities, community health focuses, unsupported careful offices, nursing homes, school-or school-based offices, modern settings, and remedial frameworks. PAs are consistently engaged with group-based models of patient care due to their relationship with physician bosses. It has been discovered to be practical for PAs to do obligations that physicians can perform, for example, preventive healthcare guiding. PAs may have the additional time accessible to go through with patients when contrasted and their physician bosses.

14.6.3 Challenges/Future Opportunities

Unmistakably the requirement for highly qualified essential care suppliers is insufficient to fulfill current needs, and future necessities will probably rise. PAs are well qualified and highly prepared to help coherence and admittance to care in a demonstrated, savvy model. PAs will probably be vital participants in gathering essential care needs. A likely role for PAs, which could be encouraged by improvements to preparing and practice strategy, would be in the plan, usage, and bearing of the conveyance of care in centers and offices the whole way across the nation using a patient-focused clinical home model (American Academy of Physician Assistants, 2008).

Chapter 15

Video

Lectures

1) **Economic analysis for health policy**

    1 hour 01 minute 53 seconds

    https://youtu.be/VxZvItklFXg

2) **Modelling and discounting in health economics**

    1 hour 42 minute 28 seconds

https://youtu.be/npQERcFOTmI

3) **Health quality and outcomes summary**

   1 hour 06 minute 55 seconds

   https://youtu.be/C5jHsjLpqDE

4) **Concept of sugar tax in health economics**

   10 minutes 04 seconds

   https://youtu.be/C5jHsjLpqDE

5) **Basics of statistics in management**

   40 minutes 25 seconds

   https://youtu.be/P1qP3er2UUM

6) **Affordable healthcare**

   1 hour 03 minute 54 seconds

   https://youtu.be/3_5GBJygWNM

HeartBeatsz

LEARNING YOUR WAY

Heartbeatsz.com

Chapter 16

References

- Abbott, A. 1988. The System of Professions: An Essay on the Division of Expert Labor. Chicago: University of Chicago Press.
- Akers, R. L. 1968. "The Professional Association and the Legal Regulation of Practice." Law and Society Review (3): 463-82.
- Agency for Healthcare Research and Quality

- (AHRQ). (n.d.). Never events. Retrieved from http://www.psnet.ahrq.gov/primer.aspx?primerID=3
- Accreditation Council for Pharmacy Education. Accreditation standards and guidelines for the professional program in pharmacy leading to the doctor of pharmacy degree. www.acpe-accredit.org/pdf/ACPE_ Revised_PharmD_Standards_Adopted_Jan152006.DOC.
- Amabile, T., Fisher, C. M., & Pillemer, J. (2014). IDEO's culture of helping. Harvard Business Review, 92, 54–61.
- American Dental Association. Dentistry—the model profession. www.ada.org/sections/about/pdfs/statements_dentistry.pdf.
- American Academy of Physician Assistants. 2008 AAPA physician assistant census report. www.aapa.org/images/stories/2008 aapacensusnationalreport.pdf.
- Becker, B. E., Huselid, M. A., & Ulrich, D. (2001). The HR scorecard: Linking people, strategy, and performance.
- Begun, J., and R. Lippincott. 1993. Strategic Adaptation in the Health Professions. San Francisco: Jossey-Bass.
- Bureau of Labor Statistics (BLS). (2014e). Physicians and surgeons. Occupational outlook handbook, 2014–15 edition. Retrieved from http://www.bls.gov/ooh/healthcare/physicians-and-surgeons.htm
- Bureau of Labor Statistics (BLS). (2014f). Physician assistants. Occupational outlook handbook, 2014–15 edition. Retrieved from http://www.bls.gov/ooh/healthcare/physician-assistants.htm
- Bureau of Labor Statistics (BLS). (2014h). Registered Nurses. Occupational outlook handbook, 2014-15 edition. Retrieved from http://www.bls.gov/ooh/healthcare/registered-nurses.htm.
- Boston, MA: Harvard Business School Press. Boblitz, M., & Thompson, J. M. (2005). Assessing the feasibility of developing centers of excellence: Six initial steps. Healthcare Financial Management, 59, 72–84.
- Broscio, M., & Scherer, J. (2003). Building job security: Strategies for becoming a highly valued contributor.

Journal of Healthcare Management, 48, 147–151.
- Buchbinder, S. B., & Thompson, J. M. (2010). Career opportunities in health care management: Perspectives from the field. Sudbury, MA: Jones and Bartlett.
- Bureau of Labor Statistics (BLS). (2014). Occupational outlook handbook 2014 edition. Retrieved from www.bls.gov/oco/ocos014.htm
- Burt, T. (2005). Leadership development as a corporate strategy: Using talent reviews to improve senior management. Healthcare Executive, 20, 14–18.
- Curtright, J. W., Stolp-Smith, S. C., & Edell, E. S. (2000). Strategic management: Development of a performance measurement system at the Mayo Clinic. Journal of Healthcare Management, 45, 58–68.
- Commission on Collegiate Nursing Education. Procedures for accreditation of baccalaureate and graduate degree nursing programs. www.aacn.nche.edu/accreditation/pdf/Procedures.pdf.
- Cervero, R. M. 1989. "Professional Practice, Learning and Continuing Education: An Integrated Perspective." PERN. 10-13.
- Dhar, M., Griffin, M., Hollin, I., & Kachnowski, S. (2012). Innovation spaces: Six strategies to inform health care. The Health Care Manager, 31, 166–177.
- Drucker, P. F. (2005). Managing oneself. Harvard Business Review, 83(1), 100–109.
- Duffy, J. R., & Lemieux, K. G. (1995, Fall). A cardiac service line approach to patient-centered care. Nursing Administration Quarterly, 20, 12–23.
- Ditlopo, Prudence, Duane Blaauw, Laetitia C. Rispel, Steve Thomas, and Posy Bidwell. "Policy implementation and financial incentives for nurses in South Africa: a case study on the occupation-specific dispensation." Global health action 6 (2013).
- John Meyer, (2011) The Complete Guide to Strategic Marketing for the Cardiovascular Service Line is published by Health Leaders Media.
- Hyde, J. C., and M. D. Fottler. 1995. "Determinants of Rural Hospital Utilization of Multiskilled Health

- Practitioners." Health Services Management Review 8 (1): 64-72.
- Emanuel, E. J. 1991. The Ends of Human Life: Medical Ethics in a Liberal Polity. Cambridge, Mass.: Harvard University Press.
- Field, M. G. 1993. "Physician in the Commonwealth of Independent States: The Difficult Passage from Bureaucrat to Professional." In The Changing Medical Profession: An International Perspective edited by E W. Hafferty and J. B. McKinlay, 162-71. New York: Oxford University Press.
- Forgotson, E. H., R. Roemer, and R. W. Newman. "Licensure of Physicians." In Report of the National Advisory Commission on Health Manpower. Washington, D.C.: U.S. Government Printing Office.
- Fernandez-Araoz, C. (2014). 21st century talent spotting. Harvard Business Review, 92(6), 46–56.
- Finley, F. R., Ivanitskaya, L. V., & Kennedy, M. H. (2007). Mentoring junior healthcare administrators: A description of mentoring practices in 127 U.S. hospitals. Journal of Healthcare Management, 52, 260–270.
- Freidson, E. 1970. Profession Of Medicine: A Study of the Sociology ofApplied Knowledge. New York: Dodd Mead.
- Freidson, E. 1994. Professionalism Reborn: Theory, Prophecy and Policy. 184-98. Chicago: University of Chicago Press
- Freedman, M. 1976. Labor Markets: Segments and Shelters. Montclair, N. Mex.: Allanheld, Osmun.
- Garman, A. N. (2010). Leadership development in the interdisciplinary context. In B. Freshman, L. Rubino, and Y. R. Chassiakos, (Eds.), Collaboration across the disciplines in health care (pp. 43–63). Sudbury, MA: Jones and Bartlett.
- Garman, A. N., McAlearney, A. S., Harrison, M. I., Song, P. H., & McHugh, M. (2011). High-performance work systems in health care management, Part 1: Development of an evidence-informed model. Health Care Management Review, 36(3), 201–213.
- Ginter, P. M., Swayne, L. E., & Duncan, W. J. (2002).

Strategic management of healthcare organizations (4th ed.). Malden, MA: Blackwell.
- Griffith, J. R. (2000). Championship management for healthcare organizations. Journal of Healthcare Management, 45, 17–31.
- Griffith, J. R. (2009). Finding the frontier of hospital management. Journal of Healthcare Management, 54(1), 57–73.
- Geretis, M. 1993. "What Patients Really Want." Health Management Quarterly (Third Quarter) 1-6.
- Johnson K. Meeting Healthy People 2010 Objective 1.7 in ASAHP programs. J Allied Health 2010;39(3):150–5.
- Hamel, G. (2007). The future of management. Boston, MA: Harvard Business School Press.
- Harrington, H. J., & Voehl, F. (2010). Innovation in health care. International Journal of Innovation Science, 2, 13–27.
- Hafferty, E W., and J. B. McKinlay, eds. 1993. The Changing Medical Profession: An International Perspective. New York: Oxford University Press.
- Huselid, M. A., Beatty, R. W., & Becker, B. E. (2005, December). "A players" or "A" positions? The strategic logic of workforce management. Harvard Business Review, 83, 100–117.
- Hyde, J. C., and M. D. Fottler. 1995. "Determinants of Rural Hospital Utilization of Multiskilled Health Practitioners." Health Services Management Review 8 (1): 64-72.
- Katz, R. L. (1974). Skills of an effective administrator. Harvard Business Review, 52, 90–102.
- Kotzee, T. J., and I. D. Couper. "What interventions do South African qualified doctors think will retain them in rural hospitals of the Limpopo province of South Africa." Rural Remote Health 6, no. 3 (2006): 581.
- Kim, T. H., & Thompson, J. M. (2012). Organizational and market factors associated with leadership development programs in hospitals: A national study. Journal of Healthcare Management, 57(2), 113–132.
- Kubica, A. J. (2008). Transitioning middle managers. Healthcare Executive, 23, 58–60.
- Landry, A. Y., & Bewley, L. W. (2010). Leadership

development, succession planning and mentoring. In S. R. Hernandez & S. J. O'Connor (Eds.), Strategic management of human resources in health services organizations (3rd ed., pp. 133–146). Clifton Park, NY: Delmar.
- Lombardi, D. M., & Schermerhorn, J. R. (2007). Healthcare management. Hoboken, NJ: John Wiley.
- Longest, B. B., Rakich, J. S., & Darr, K. (2000). Managing health services organizations and systems. Baltimore, MD: Health Professions Press.
- Maccoby, M., Norman, C. L., Norman, C. J., & Margolies, R. (2013). Transforming health care leadership: A systems guide to improve patient care, decrease costs, and improve population health. San Francisco: CA: Jossey-Bass.
- McLaughlin, C. P., and A. D. Kaluzny. 1990. "Total Quality Management in Health: Making it Work." Health Care Management Review 15 (3): 7-14.
- McAlearney, A. S. (2005). Exploring mentoring and leadership development in health care organizations: Experience and opportunities. Career Development International, 10(6/7), 493–511.
- McAlearney, A. S. (2008). Using leadership development programs to improve quality and efficiency in healthcare. Journal of Healthcare Management, 53(5), 319–332.
- McAlearney, A. S. (2010). Executive leadership development in U.S. health systems. Journal of Healthcare Management, 55(3), 206–224.
- McAlearney, A. S., Robbins, J., Garman, A. N., & Song, P. H. (2013). Implementing high performance work practices in healthcare organizations: Qualitative and conceptual evidence. Journal of Healthcare Management, 58(6), 446–462.
- McHugh, M., Garman, A., McAlearney, A., Song, P., & Harrison, M. (2010). Using workforce practices to drive quality improvement: A guide for hospitals. Rockville, MD: Agency for Healthcare Research and Quality. Retrieved from www.hret.org/workforce/resources/workforce-guide.pdf
- National Center for Healthcare Leadership (NCHL).

(2010). Best practices in healthcare leadership academies. Chicago, IL: Author. Retrieved from http://www.nchl.org/Documents/Ctrl_Hyperlink/doccopy5381_uid6102014456192.pdf
- National Academies Press. Training physicians for public health careers. books.nap.edu/openbook.php?record_id11915&page29.
- Ogden, G. (2010). Talent management in a time of cost management. Healthcare Financial Management, 64(3), 80–82, 84.
- Pieper, S. K. (2005). Reading the right signals: How to strategically manage with scorecards. Healthcare Executive, 20, 9–14.
- Philip Kotler and Roberta N. Clarke, (1987).Marketing for Health Care Organizations (Englewood Cliffs, NJ: Prentice Hall.
- Parsons, M. L., and C. L. Murdaugh. 1994. Patient-Centered Care: A Model For Restructuring. Rockville, Md.: Aspen Publishers.
- Rollins, G. (2003). Succession planning: Laying the foundation for smooth transitions and effective leaders. Healthcare Executive, 18, 14–18.
- Ross, A., Wenzel, F. J., & Mitlyng, J. W. (2002). Leadership for the future: Core competencies in health care. Chicago, IL: Health Administration Press/AUPHA Press.
- Scott, G. (2009). The leader as coach. Healthcare Executive, 24(4), 40–43.
- Scott, T., Mannion, R., Davies, H. T. O., & Marshall, M. M. (2003). Implementing culture change in health care: Theory and practice. International Journal for Quality in Health Care. Retrieved from http://intqhc.oxfordjournals.org/content/15/2/111
- Schon, D. 1983. The Reflective Practitioner: How Professionals Think in Action. Basic Books.
- Squazzo, J. D. (2009, November/December). Cultivating tomorrow's leaders: Comprehensive development strategies ensure continued success. Healthcare Executive, 24(6), 8–20.
- Staren, E. D., Braun, D. P., & Denny, D. (2010). Optimizing innovation in health care organizations.

Physician Executive Journal, March/April, 54–62.
- Studer, Q. (2003). Hardwiring excellence. Gulf Breeze, FL: Fire Starter.
- Schneller, E. S., P. Hood-Szivek, and R. G. Hughes. 1994. "The Future of Medicine." In The Physician Executive, 2d ed., edited by W. Curry. Tampa, Fla.: The American College of Physician Executives.
- The Economist, 1994. "Why Doctors?" 10 December.
- Torpey, E. (2014, Spring). Healthcare: Millions of jobs now and in the future. Occupational Outlook Quarterly. Retrieved from http://www.bls.gov/careeroutlook/2014/spring/art03.pdf
- Thompson, J. M. (2007). Health services administration. In S. Chisolm (Ed.), The health professions: Trends and opportunities in U.S. health care (pp. 357–372). Sudbury, MA: Jones and Bartlett.
- Thompson, J. M. (2010). Understanding and managing organizational change: Implications for public health management. Journal of Public Health Management & Practice, 16(20), 167–173.
- Thompson, J. M., & Kim, T. H. (2013). A profile of hospitals with leadership development programs. The Health Care Manager, 32(2), 179–188.
- Thompson, J. M., & Temple, A. (2015). Early careerist interest and participation in leadership development programs. The Health Care Manager, 34(4), 350–358.
- Vujicic, Marko, and Pascal Zurn. "The dynamics of the health labour market." The International journal of health planning and management 21, no. 2 (2006): 101-115.
- Vaidya, A. (2013, June 18). Survey: Number of hospital-employed physicians up 6%. Becker's Hospital Review. Retrieved from http://www.beckershospitalreview.com/hospital-physicianrelationships/survey-number-of-hospital-employed-physicians-up-6.html
- Wolinsky, F. 1993. "The Professional Dominance, Deprofessionalization, Proletarianization, and Corporatization Perspectives: An Overview and Synthesis." In The ChangingMedica1Profmion: An International Perspective edited by F. W. Hafferty and J.

B. McKinlay, 11-24. New York: Oxford University Press.

Time to Practice

Questions

Chapter 1:
1: Who is responsible for coordinating healthcare aspects?

1. Healthcare workers
2. Healthcare directors
3. Healthcare practitioner
4. Healthcare managers

2: Who maintains and collects the patient health data?

1. IT experts
2. Healthcare workers
3. Coding experts
4. All of above

3: Who collaborate with cybersecurity experts to ensure that the database is safe?

1. Healthcare information manager
2. Assisted living administrator
3. Healthcare quality improvement manager
4. Hospice administrator

4: Inpatient and outpatient care facilities need administrators for improving roles in:

- Outpatient settings
- Doctor practices
- Both 1 and 2
- None of above

Chapter 2:

1: Which statement is not true about healthcare management?

- They are in charge of the whole healthcare organization.
- They determine if another representative is required.

- They are in charge of the corporate side of healthcare organizations.
- They determine the best methods for assisting employees.

2: Which statement is not true about healthcare administration?
- They understand office's treatment.
- Determine how each division should be run.
- Focus on hospital needs
- Head of healthcare organizations.

3: What is similar in both healthcare management and administration?
- Both implement innovations and strategies.
- Both focus on hospital needs
- Both manage the healthcare organizations
- Both helps employees

Chapter 3:

1: Which of the following type is not external domains?

- Accreditation
- Competitors
- Licensure
- Financial performance

2: Which of the following type is not internal domains?

- Budgeting
- Patient satisfaction
- Community demographics
- Technology acquisitions

3: why associations are formed?

- To manage staff
- To achieve goals
- To set scope
- To perform critical tasks

4: Manager should think about which domain while making decisions?

- Internal
- External
- Both
- None of the above

Chapter 4:

1: After completing the management cycle managers develop how many management capacities?

- Six
- Two
- Seven
- Ten

2: in designing, what a manager job entails?

- establishing a direction
- Implementations of goals.
- determining requirements
- All of the above

3: Rational skills enable the manager to?

- Communicate with workers
- Communicate with colleagues
- Both 1 and 2
- Communicate with boss

4: Which skills have the ability to fundamentally break down and address difficult problem?

- Management skills
- Rational skills
- Academic skills
- None of the above

Chapter 5:

1: What are some managerial roles positions?

- Line manager positions
- Records manager positions
- Staff manager positions
- Both 1 and 3

2: Which one is not the duty of the staff manager?

- complete work
- motivate their subordinates
- routinely supervise others
- None of the above

3: In hierarchical architecture which structure is the most critical one?

- Large organizations
- Small organizations
- Medium organizations
- Manageable organizations

4: What is management's main focus?

- effective health-care management
- exercising professional judgment and skills
- administrative capacities Within a unit/group
- All of the above

Chapter 6:
1: Following are the guidelines of the code of conduct for an organization except?

- Vision
- Qualities
- Control
- mission

2: To achieve execution, one must value the benefits of identifying and achieving goals and priorities for the unit/service and organization's work this called?

- High management
- High execution
- High results
- High organization

3: Each company has its own distinct culture, which is defined by?

- shared mentalities
- shared convictions
- behaviors of its employees
- All of the above

4: Educational mediations and skill-building exercises aimed at strengthening people's leadership skills are referred to as?

- Organization development
- Skills development
- Leadership development
- None of the above

Chapter 7:

1: Are managers and leaders the same?

- Yes
- No
- Not necessarily
- None of the above

2: Managers priority is to?

- People
- Results
- Organization
- Work

3: Leaders focus on?

- Transactional
- Transformational
- Both 1 and 2
- None of the above

4: Mangers teams include?

- Managers
- Subordinates
- Followers
- Workers

Chapter 8:

1: Kaiser Permanente model is used in?
- Organizing results
- Managing orders
- Administration of population's size
- Maintaining discipline

2: The new procedures of reshaping work's dependent on such investigations may weaken the?
- Work orientation
- Action orientation
- Both 1 and 2
- None of the above

3: Which article has recommended that "the fate of specialists looks grim"?
- The workers
- The people
- The Economist's
- None of the above

4: The person who identify that the satisfaction of the patient have prolonged effects on their organization's feasibility is a?
- Worker
- Manager
- Leader
- Staff

Chapter 9:

1: SOP is a short form of?

- System operational procedure
- System of productivity
- System of the profession
- Both 1 and 3

2: Strategic decision making includes?

- Narrative itself is changed as it becomes appropriated
- Experience is used to inform and legitimize
- Perceived POSs are reconsidered
- All of the above

3: Which idea of Freidson's deals with rebuilding the medical services working environment and expert work?

- somewhat crude and bureaucratic
- bureaucratic labor market
- Both 1 and 2
- None of the above

4: The term gatekeeper is used for?

- Workers
- Doctors
- Researchers
- Managers

Chapter 10:

1: The standards of health care morals are?

- Helpfulness
- non-maleficence
- Autonomy and equity
- All of the above

2: Non-Maleficence means?

- To work perfectly
- To manage better
- To do no damage
- To help others

3: What does National Association for Healthcare Quality suggests about an in-house health care quality professional manages better?

- Work ethics
- Organization skills
- Work environment
- Moral culture

4: The law of shields representatives from provocation because of sex, shading, or identity is?

- The Equal Opportunity Employment Committee
- The safety Act
- The Civil Rights Act
- None of the above

Chapter 11:

1: What is fundamental to a successful healthcare system?

- Human resources
- Finance department
- Quality check
- Records keeping

2: Negative feedback was received from their ?

- Coworkers
- Supervisors
- Friends
- None of the above

3: Salary increases may not be feasible in?

- Eastern countries
- High resource country
- Low resource country
- All of the above

4: It's important to follow positive management guidelines and have quality supervision. This can be accomplished by enhancing?

- Workers
- Quality control
- Results production
- Management efficiency

Chapter 12:

1: What is constantly evolving because of technical advances or government orders?

- Healthcare industry
- Food industry
- Transport industry
- Internet services

2: What does Healthcare Strategic Planning entails?

- Getting results
- Faster work
- Setting priorities
- Managing

3: In Healthcare Strategic Planning you have to set targets according too?

- Current economic conditions
- Government policies
- Technical advances
- All of the above

4: In healthcare management, effective preparation will help you build?

- Transparency
- Enhance communication
- Both 1 and 2
- None of the above

Chapter 13:

1: When was marketing introduced into healthcare field?

- 1970
- 1960
- 1982
- 1980

2: Production depends upon?

- Reliable services
- Efficient services
- Both 1 and 2
- None of the above

3: The marketing philosophy is centered on?

- Worker's availability
- Costumers needs
- Efficient results
- All of the above

4: What are the elements of comprehensive marketing?

- Integrated marketing
- Relationship marketing
- Success marketing
- All of the above

Chapter 14:

1: Health care associations have many clinical, administrative, and uphold experts to convey health care services to their?

- Workers
- Bosses
- Patients
- Supervisors

2: Allied health includes?

- Dietetics
- Athletic preparing
- Occupational and physical therapy
- All of the above

3: The assessment, diagnosis, prevention, and additionally treatment of illnesses and disorders of oral cavity are called?

- Dentistry
- Preventive measures
- Both 1 and 2
- None of the above

4: In healthcare field who survey a patient's wellbeing, give clinical treatment, and teach patients and families?

- Doctors
- Nurses
- Receptionists
- Interns

Time to Practice

Answers

Chapter 1:

1: Who is responsible for coordinating healthcare aspects?

- Healthcare workers
- Healthcare directors
- Healthcare practitioner (Correct)
- Healthcare managers

2: Who maintains and collects the patient health data?

- IT experts
- Healthcare workers
- Coding experts
- All of above (correct)

3: Who collaborate with cybersecurity experts to ensure that the

database is safe?
- Healthcare information manager (correct)
- Assisted living administrator
- Healthcare quality improvement manager
- Hospice administrator

4: Inpatient and outpatient care facilities need administrators for improving roles in:
- Outpatient settings
- Doctor practices
- Both 1 and 2 (correct)
- None of above

Chapter 2:

1: Which statement is not true about healthcare management?
- They are in charge of the whole healthcare organization.
- They determine if another representative is required.
- They are in charge of the corporate side of healthcare organizations.
- They determine the best methods for assisting employees. (correct)

2: Which statement is not true about healthcare administration?
- They understand office's treatment.
- Determine how each division should be run.
- Focus on hospital needs
- Head of healthcare organizations. (correct)

3: What is similar in both healthcare management and

administration?

- Both implement innovations and strategies. (correct)
- Both focus on hospital needs
- Both manage the healthcare organizations
- Both helps employees

Chapter 3:

1: Which of the following type is not external domains?

- Accreditation
- Competitors
- Licensure
- Financial performance (correct)

2: Which of the following type is not internal domains?

- Budgeting
- Patient satisfaction
- Community demographics (correct)
- Technology acquisitions

3: why associations are formed?

- To manage staff
- To achieve goals (correct)
- To set scope
- To perform critical tasks

4: Manager should think about which domain while making decisions?

- Internal
- External

- Both (correct)
- None of the above

Chapter 4:

1: After completing the management cycle managers develop how many management capacities?

- Six (correct)
- Two
- Seven
- Ten

2: in designing, what, manager jobs entail too?

- establishing a direction
- Implementations of goals.
- determining requirements
- All of the above (correct)

3: Rational skills enable the manager to?

- Communicate with workers
- Communicate with colleagues
- Both 1 and 2 (correct)
- Communicate with boss

4: Which skills have the ability to fundamentally break down and address difficult problem?

- Management skills
- Rational skills
- Academic skills (correct)
- None of the above

Chapter 5:

1: What are some managerial roles positions?

- Line manager positions
- Records manager positions
- Staff manager positions
- Both 1 and 3 (correct)

2: Which one is not the duty of the staff manager?

- complete work
- motivate their subordinates
- routinely supervise others (correct)
- None of the above

3: In hierarchical architecture which structure is the most critical one?

- Large organizations (correct)
- Small organizations
- Medium organizations
- Manageable organizations

4: What is management's main focus?

- effective health-care management
- exercising professional judgment and skills
- administrative capacities Within a unit/group
- All of the above (correct)

Chapter 6:

1: Following are the guidelines of the code of conduct for an organization except?

- Vision
- Qualities
- Control (correct)
- mission

2: To achieve execution, one must value the benefits of identifying and achieving goals and priorities for the unit/service and organization's work this called?

- High management
- High execution (correct)
- High results
- High organization

3: Each company has its own distinct culture, which is defined by?

- shared mentalities
- shared convictions
- behaviors of its employees
- All of the above (correct)

4: Educational mediations and skill-building exercises aimed at strengthening people's leadership skills are referred to as?

- Organization development
- Skills development
- Leadership development (correct)
- None of the above

Chapter 7:

1: Are managers and leaders the same?

- Yes
- No
- Not necessarily (correct)
- None of the above

2: Manager's priority is to?

- People
- Results
- Organization
- Work (correct)

3: Leaders focus on?

- Transactional
- Transformational (correct)
- Both 1 and 2
- None of the above

4: Mangers teams include?

- Managers
- Subordinates (correct)
- Followers
- Workers

Chapter 8:

1: Kaiser Permanente model is used in?
- Organizing results
- Managing orders
- Administration of population's size (correct)
- Maintaining discipline

2: The new procedures of reshaping work's dependent on such investigations may weaken the?
- Work orientation
- Action orientation (correct)
- Both 1 and 2
- None of the above

3: Which article has recommended that "the fate of specialists looks grim"?
- The workers
- The people
- The Economist's (correct)
- None of the above

4: The person who identify that the satisfaction of the patient have prolonged effects on their organization's feasibility is a?
- Worker
- Manager (correct)
- Leader
- Staff

Chapter 9:

1: SOP is a short form of?

- System operational procedure
- System of productivity
- System of the profession (correct)
- Both 1 and 3

2: Strategic decision making includes?

- Narrative itself is changed as it becomes appropriated
- Experience are used to inform and legitimize
- Perceived POSs are reconsidered
- All of the above (correct)

3: Which idea of Freidson's deals with rebuilding the medical services working environment and expert work?

- somewhat crude and bureaucratic
- bureaucratic labor market (correct)
- Both 1 and 2
- None of the above

4: The term gatekeeper is used for?

- Workers
- Doctors (correct)
- Researchers
- Managers

Chapter 10:

1: The standards of health care morals are?

- Helpfulness
- non-maleficence
- Autonomy and equity
- All of the above (correct)

2: Non-Maleficence means?

- To work perfectly
- To manage better
- To do no damage (correct)
- To help others

3: What does National Association for Healthcare Quality suggests about an in-house health care quality professional manages better?

- Work ethics
- Organization skills
- Work environment
- Moral culture (correct)

4: The law of shields representatives from provocation because of sex, shading, or identity is?

- The Equal Opportunity Employment Committee
- The safety Act
- The Civil Rights Act (correct)
- None of the above

Chapter 11:

1: What is fundamental to a successful healthcare system?

- Human resources (correct)
- Finance department
- Quality check
- Records keeping

2: Negative feedback was received from their?

- Coworkers
- Supervisors (correct)
- Friends
- None of the above

3: Salary increases may not be feasible in?

- Eastern countries
- High resource country
- Low resource country (correct)
- All of the above

4: It's important to follow positive management guidelines and have quality supervision. This can be accomplished by enhancing?

- Workers
- Quality control
- Results production
- Management efficiency (correct)

Chapter 12:

1: What is constantly evolving because of technical advances or government orders?

- Healthcare industry (correct)
- Food industry
- Transport industry
- Internet services

2: What does Healthcare Strategic Planning entails?

- Getting results
- Faster work
- Setting priorities (correct)
- Managing

3: In Healthcare Strategic Planning you have to set targets according too?

- Current economic conditions
- Government policies
- Technical advances
- All of the above (correct)

4: In healthcare management, effective preparation will help you build?

- Transparency
- Enhance communication
- Both 1 and 2 (correct)
- None of the above

Chapter 13:

1: When was marketing introduced into healthcare field?

- 1970
- 1960
- 1982
- 1980 (correct)

2: Production depends upon?

- Reliable services
- Efficient services
- Both 1 and 2 (correct)
- None of the above

3: The marketing philosophy is centered on?

- Worker's availability
- Costumers needs (correct)
- Efficient results
- All of the above

4: What are the elements of comprehensive marketing?

- Integrated marketing
- Relationship marketing
- Success marketing
- All of the above (correct)

Chapter 14:

1: Health care associations have many clinical, administrative, and uphold experts to convey health care services to their?

- Workers
- Bosses
- Patients (correct)
- Supervisors

2: Allied health includes?

- Dietetics
- Athletic preparing
- Occupational and physical therapy
- All of the above (correct)

3: The assessment, diagnosis, prevention, and additionally treatment of illnesses and disorders of oral cavity are called?

- Dentistry (correct)
- Preventive measures
- Both 1 and 2
- None of the above

4: In healthcare field who survey a patient's wellbeing, give clinical treatment, and teach patients and families?

- Doctors
- Nurses (correct)
- Receptionists
- Interns

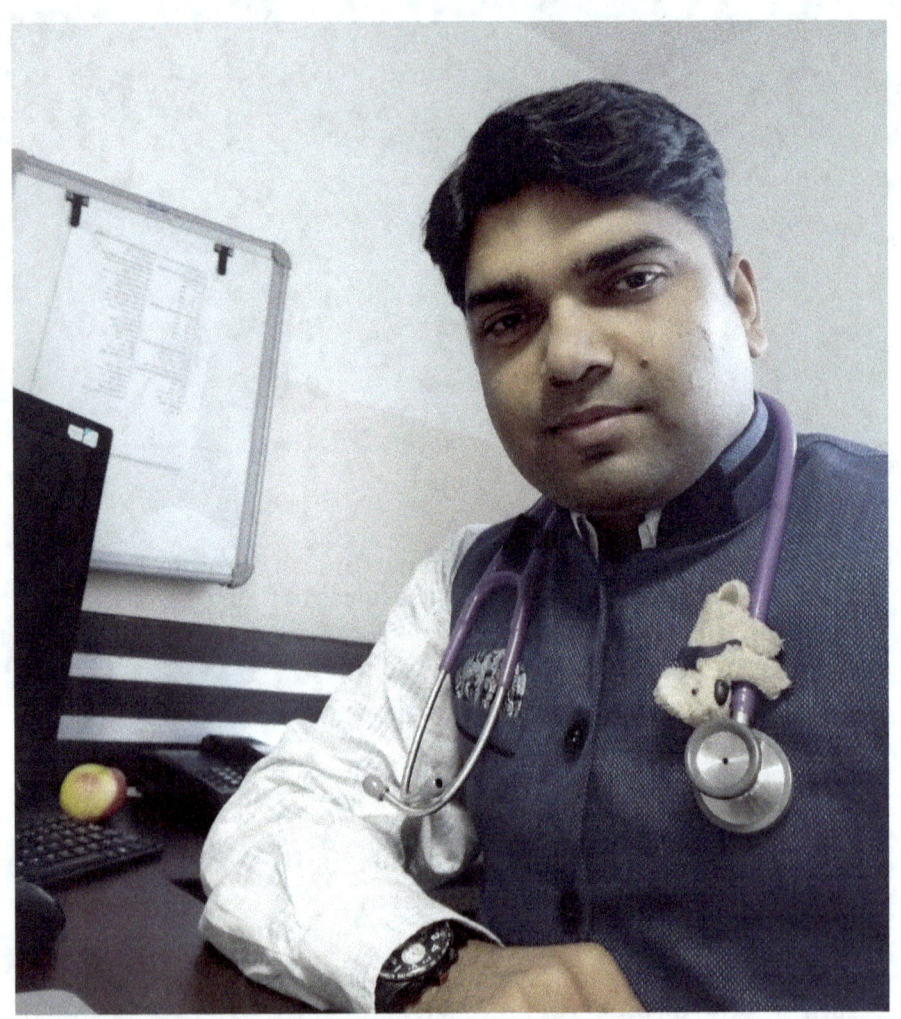

Brief biodata

Dr Narendra Kumar is European Board-Certified Cardiac electrophysiologist (ECES) with his doctorate thesis in cardiology on

Atrial fibrillation ablation from Maastricht University Medical Centre, Netherlands (ranked among top 50 clinical university of world). He is also a program chair for an International Cardiology program and visiting Professor- Cardiology for Edu University (Germany, Slovenia and Malta).

His primary interest lies in atrial fibrillation, arrhythmia management, Heart failure and cardiovascular economics. He has extensive experience with >3500 ablation procedures and devices implantation (CRT, AICD, Wireless & His bundle pacemaker and Complex pacemakers) with >70 publications in reputed journals including JACC and Heart rhythm journal. He has >12 years of experience in Cardiology.

He was awarded "NRI of the year award" 2018 for academics by Times group. He also received American Heart rhythm Society scholarship 2018 for advance heart arrhythmia training at St Luke's medical center, USA. He received American College of Cardiology 2019 travel award. He was trained earlier at some of the best hospitals across USA, UK, Germany and Netherlands.

He is a Fellow of

1] Royal college of Physicians, Edinburg UK (FRCP)

2] European Society of Cardiology (FESC)

3] American college of Cardiology (FACC)

His 2 papers including "ATSCA study" has been referenced in 2017 expert consensus on atrial fibrillation ablation guidelines. He has also worked as a reviewer for journals such as The Lancet and global consultant for various studies as Discovery, painfree-sst and improveSCA. He graduated in Health economics and cardiovascular management from London School of economics. He is "International Education Tutor" and also member of European Society of Cardiology task force groups.

He is also responsible for approval of "World's first catheter for epicardial ventricular tachycardia ablation" from TGA for Abbott (USA). He is currently working at Manchester University Hospital. He is a visiting faculty and "teacher of teachers" at various global academic cardiology hospitals globally.

The woods are lovely, dark and deep,
But I have promises to keep,
And miles to go before I sleep,
And miles to go before I sleep.

- ROBERT FROST.

www.ingramcontent.com/pod-product-compliance
Lightning Source LLC
Chambersburg PA
CBHW050057230526

45470CB00004B/1572